PLAB 1
Revision Book

Extended Matching Questions
and
Single Best Answer Questions

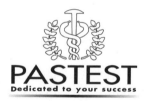

PASTEST
Dedicated to your success

Dedication

I would like to dedicate this book to my parents, Dr. Rudra Bahan Chatterjee and Dr. Sutapa Chatterjee, whose constant encouragement and guidance has helped me to be what I am today. I also want to thank my wife, Mrs. Anuradha Chatterjee, for patiently supporting me throughout this project.

Acknowledgement

We are most grateful to Dr Stephen Waring (Consultant Physician in Acute Medicine and Toxicology) for his help with this project.

PLAB 1
Revision Book

Extended Matching Questions
and
Single Best Answer Questions

J. Chatterjee MBBS, DFFP, DRCOG
Registrar in Obstetrics and Gynaecology
Walsgrave Hospital
University Hospitals of Coventry and Warwickshire
Coventry

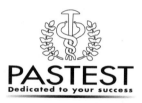

PASTEST
Dedicated to your success

© 2004 PASTEST Ltd
Egerton Court
Parkgate Estate
Knutsford
Cheshire
WA16 8DX

Telephone: 01565 752000

First published 2004

ISBN: 1 904 62717 X

A catalogue record for this book is available from the British Library.

The information contained within this book was obtained by the authors from
reliable sources. However, while every effort has been made to ensure its
accuracy, no responsibility for loss, damage or injury occasioned to any person
acting or refraining from action as a result of information contained herein can
be accepted by the publishers or authors.

PasTest Revision Books and Intensive Courses

PasTest has been established in the field of postgraduate medical education
since 1972, providing revision books and intensive study courses for doctors
preparing for their professional examinations. Books and courses are available
for the following specialties:

**MRCGP, MRCP Part 1 and 2, MRCPCH Part 1 and 2, MRCPsych, MRCS,
MRCOG, DRCOG, DCH, FRCA, PLAB.**

For further details contact:

PasTest, Freepost, Knutsford, Cheshire WA16 7BR
Tel: 01565 752000 Fax: 01565 650264
www.pastest.co.uk enquiries@pastest.co.uk

Cover design by Recognition
Text prepared by Vision Typesetting Ltd, Manchester
Printed and bound in Great Britain by Page Bros Ltd, Norwich

Contents

Introduction

Welcome to another PLAB Part 1 preparation book. The format of this book reflects recent changes to the PLAB Part 1 examination.

The examination consists of extended matching questions (EMQs) and single best answer (SBAs) questions. The examination will last 3 hours and a there will be a total of 200 questions which are divided into a number of themes with a proportion of single best answer questions (no more than 30% of the total).

Part 1 of this book contains five chapters covering: *Surgery, Medicine, Paediatrics, Psychiatry and Obstetrics & Gynaecology* with a mixture of extended matching and single best answer questions.
Part 2 contains one practice paper of 200 questions with randomised subjects and question formats to mirror the actual examination.

Preferences for exam preparation vary – some candidates like to work through as many questions as possible and use that as a focus for subsequent revision, others pre-read subject areas and dip into question and answer books or you may wish to use this book *especially the Practice Paper* to work through 'under exam conditions' in three hours to assess your performance and progress. The timing in the examination is tight with less that one minute per question. It is useful to practice this timing. The examination is not negatively marked and failure to answer all questions is a missed opportunity.

The standard of the examination is that required to ensure successful candidates are able to perform at Senior House Officer level in the NHS. The skills tested are those achieved through study and clinical experience.

The pass mark will vary with each sitting. The minimum score for success is likely to be in the region of 63%.

Information about the PLAB test and registration in the UK can be found on the General Medical Council's website: www.gmc-uk.org.

We wish you success in your examination. Good luck.

List of Co-authors

Medicine
Raja Dhar MBBS MRCP (UK) MD
Specialist Registrar, Respiratory Medicine and G(I)M,
Sunderland Royal Hospital, Northern Deanery

Surgery
Shafiul Chowdhury MBBS MRCSI MRCS (Glas.)
Clinical Fellow in Urology, Department of Urology,
Royal Hospital of St Bartholomew and Royal London
Hospital, Barts and the London NHS Trust, London

Obstetrics and Gynaecology
Jayanta Chatterjee MBBS DFFP DRCOG
Registrar in Obstetrics and Gynaecology,
Walsgrave Hospital, University Hospitals of Coventry
and Warwickshire, Coventry

Paediatrics
Dr Abanti Paul MBBS DCH DRCOG MRCGP
General Practitioner, London

Psychiatry
Dr Rahul Bhattacharya MBBS DPM
Senior House Officer in Vincent Square Eating Disorder
Unit, Charing Cross Psychiatric Rotation, London

Preface

Congratulations to the team of authors for writing this excellent book of practice papers for the PLAB examination. With its exhaustive set of EMQs and SBAs, it has a very user-friendly structure, designed to enhance deep learning. As the PLAB exam aims to test core knowledge across the whole curriculum, the book will prove to be not only a study book for doctors sitting the examination itself, but is also a very helpful preparatory book for final year medical students.

Extended Matching Questions and Single Best Answers test a deeper level of knowledge than can be tested in the traditional MCQ format. This helps to get around an important disadvantage of MCQs, which have a tendency to test only superficial factual knowledge.

I am sure that this book will be good value for money and will enhance the ability of readers to learn deeply. In the words of Hippocrates "The life so short, the craft so long to learn".

Mr Laurence Wood FRCS FRCOG
Associate Post-Graduate Dean, West-Midlands Deanery, Consultant Obstetrician & Gynaecologist, Walsgrave Hospital, Coventry

List of Abbreviations

A&E	Accident and Emergency (department)
AAA	aortic abdominal aneurysm
ABC	airway, breathing, circulation
ABPA	allergic bronchopulmonary aspergillosis
ABPI	ankle-brachial pressure index
ACE	angiotensin-converting enzyme
ACEI	angiotensin-converting enzyme inhibitor
aCL	anticardiolipin
ACTH	adrenocorticotrophic hormone
ADHD	attention-deficit hyperactive disorder
AF	atrial fibrillation
AFI	amniotic fluid index
AIDS	acquired immunodeficiency syndrome
ALP	alkaline phosphatase
α_1-AT	α_1-antitrypsin
AMA	antimitochondrial antibody
AN	anorexia nervosa
ANA	antinuclear antibody
apo	apolipoprotein
APP	amyloid precursor protein
APS	antiphospholipid syndrome
APTT	activated partial thromboplastin time
APUD	amine precursor uptake and decarboxylation
AST	aspartate aminotransferase
ATLS	Advanced Trauma Life Support
ATN	acute tubular necrosis
AUDIT	Alcohol-Use Disorders Identification Test
AXR	abdominal X-ray
bd	*bis die* (= twice a day)
BDI	Beck's Depression Inventory

βHCG	beta human chorionic gonadotrophin
BMI	body mass index
BMJ	*British Medical Journal*
BNF	*British National Formulary*
BP	blood pressure
bpm	beats per minute
BTS	British Thoracic Society
BV	bacterial vaginosis
CABG	coronary artery bypass graft
CAD	coronary artery disease
CAGE	Cut down, Annoyed by criticism, Guilty about drinking, Eye-opener drinks (a test for alcoholism)
CAH	congenital adrenal hyperplasia
CAPD	continuous ambulatory peritoneal dialysis
CBT	cognitive behaviour therapy
CCF	congestive cardiac failure
CDH	congenital dysplasia of the hip
CF	cystic fibrosis
CFS	chronic fatigue syndrome
ChE	cholinesterase
CJD	Creutzfeldt–Jakob disease
CLO	*Campylobacter*-like organism (rapid urease test)
CNS	central nervous system
COPD	chronic obstructive pulmonary disease
CPK	creatinine phosphokinase
CRP	C-reactive protein
CSF	cerebrospinal fluid
CT	computed tomography
CT PA	computed tomography pulmonary angiogram
CTG	cardiotochograph
CVS	chorionic villus sampling
CXR	chest X-ray
DEXA	dual-energy X-ray absorptiometry
DIC	disseminated/diffuse intravascular coagulation
DIP	distal interphalangeal
DLE	disseminated lupus erythematosus
DMSA	dimercaptosuccinic acid
dsDNA	double-stranded DNA
DSM-4	*Diagnostic and Statistical Manual*, 4th edition

DST	dexamethasone suppression test
DT	delirium tremens
DVLA	Driver and Vehicle Licensing Agency
DVT	deep vein thrombosis
EBV	Epstein–Barr virus
ECG	electrocardiogram/graphy
ECT	electroconvulsive therapy
EGC	early gastric cancer
EMG	electromyogram/graphy
EMQs	extended matching questions
ERCP	endoscopic retrograde cholangiopancreatography
ESR	erythrocyte sedimentation rate
FBC	full blood count
FEV_1	forced expiratory volume in 1 second
FFP	fresh-frozen plasma
FNAC	fine-needle aspiration cytology
FSH	follicle-stimulating hormone
FTD	frontotemporal dementia
5-FU	5-fluorouracil
G6PD	glucose 6-phosphate dehydrogenase
GBS	group-B streptococcus; Guillain–Barré syndrome
GCS	Glasgow Coma Scale
GGT	gamma-glutamyl transferase
GHQ	General Health Questionnaire
GI	gastrointestinal
GIFT	gamete intrafallopian transfer
GMC	General Medical Council
GP	general practitioner
GUM	genitourinary medicine
h	hour
h/o	history of
Hb	haemoglobin
HB	hepatitis B
HDL	high-density lipoprotein
HIV	human immunodeficiency virus
HOCM	hypertrophic obstructive cardiomyopathy
HPV	human papillomavirus
HRCT	high-resolution computed tomography
HRT	hormone replacement therapy

HSG	hysterosalpingogram
HSP	Henoch–Schönlein purpura
HTN	hypertension
HUS	haemolytic-uraemic syndrome
HVS	high vaginal swab
Hycosy	hysterosalpingo contrast sonography
IBS	irritable bowel syndrome
ICD-10	*International Classification of Disease*, 10th edition
ICSI	intracytoplasmic sperm injection
IgG	immunoglobulin G
IHD	ischaemic heart disease
im	intramuscular
INR	international normalised ratio
IPT	interpersonal therapy
IT	information technology
ITU	intensive therapy/treatment unit
IU	international units
IUCD	intrauterine contraceptive device
IUD	intrauterine death
IUGR	intrauterine growth retardation
IUI	intrauterine insemination
iv	intravenous
IVF	*in vitro* fertilisation
IVS	interventricular septum
IVT	intravenous transfusion
IVU	intravenous urography
JVP	jugular venous pressure
kJ	kilojoule
KUB	kidney, ureter, bladder
LBD	Lewy body dementia
LDH	Lactate dehydrogenase
LDL	low-density lipoprotein
LFT	liver function test
LGV	lymphogranuloma venereum
LH	luteinising hormone
LHRH	luteinising hormone-releasing hormone
LKM	liver-kidney microsomal (antibody)
LL	lepromatous leprosy
LLETZ	large loop excision of the transformation zone

LMP	last menstrual period
LSD	lysergic diethylamide
LV	left ventricle
MAG3	mercaptoacetyl triglycine
MAI	*Mycobacterium avium intracellulare*
MAO	monoamine oxidase
MAOI	monoamine oxidase inhibitor
MCH	mean corpuscular haemoglobin
MCU	micturating cystourethrography
MCUG	micturating cystourethrogram
MCV	mean corpuscular volume
MEN	multiple endocrine neoplasia
MI	myocardial infarct/ischaemia
MIBG	metaiodobenzylguanidine (imaging)
min	minute
MMSE	Mini-Mental State Examination
MODS	multi-organ dysfunction syndrome
mph	miles per hour
MRI	magnetic resonance imaging
MSU	mid-stream urine
NAI	non-accidental injury
NASH	non-alcoholic steatohepatitis
NGU	non-gonococcal urethritis
NHS	National Health Service
NICE	National Institute for Clinical Excellence
NMS	neuroleptic malignant syndrome
NSAIDs	non-steroidal anti-inflammatory drugs
o/e	on examination
OA	osteoarthritis
OCD	obsessive-compulsive disorder
OCP	oral contraceptive pill
OGTT	oral glucose tolerance test
OHSS	ovarian hyperstimulation syndrome
OPD	outpatients department
$p(CO_2)$	partial pressure of carbon dioxide
$p(O_2)$	partial pressure of oxygen
P/A	per abdomen
P/S	presenting symptom; per speculum
P/V	per vagina

PA	pulmonary angiogram
PANSS	Positive and Negative Syndrome Scale
PAS	Periodic acid–Schiff (stain)
PCA	patient-controlled analgesia
PCOS	polycystic ovarian syndrome
PCP	*Pneumocystis carinii* pneumonia (new name *Pneumocystis jiroveci*)
PDA	patent ductus arteriosus
PDS	polydioxanone sutures
PE	pulmonary embolism
PID	pelvic inflammatory disease
PMF	progressive massive fibrosis
PMR	polymyalgia rheumatica
PN	pyelonephritis
PND	postnatal depression
POP	progesterone-only pills
PPH	postpartum haemorrhage
prn	*pro re nata* (= as required)
PSA	prostate-specific antigen
PSE	Present State Examination
PT	prothrombin time
PU	peptic ulcer
PXE	pseudoxanthoma elasticum
RA	rheumatoid arthritis
RBBB	right bundle branch block
RBC	red blood cell
RCOG	Royal College of Obstetricians and Gynaecologists
REM	random eye movement (sleep)
RDS	respiratory distress syndrome
RMO	responsible medical officer
RTA	road traffic accident
RV	right ventricle
s	second
SBAs	single best answers
sc	subcutaneous
SHBG	sex hormone-binding globulin
SLE	systemic lupus erythematosus
SSRI	selective serotonin-reuptake inhibitor

STD	sexually transmitted disease
STI	sexually transmitted infection
SUFE	slipped upper femoral epiphysis
TAS	transabdominal scan
TB	tuberculosis
TBIDA	trimethylbromoiminodiacetic acid ([^{99}Tc^m]TBIDA)
Tc	technetium
TCA	tricyclic antidepressant
[^{99}Tc^m]DMSA	technetium 99m-labelled dimercaptosuccinic acid
TFT	thyroid function test
TIA	transient ischaemic attack
TNF-α	tumour necrosis factor-alpha
TRUS	transrectal ultrasonography
TSST-1	toxic-shock syndrome toxin, type 1
TTP	thrombotic thrombocytopenic purpura
TURP	transurethral resection of the prostate
TV	*Trichomonas vaginalis*
TVT	tension-free vaginal tape
U&E	urea and electrolytes
UDP	uridine diphosphate
URTI	upper respiratory tract infection
USS	ultrasound scan
UTI	urinary tract infection
UV	ultraviolet
vCJD	variant Creutzfeldt–Jakob disease
VDRL	Venereal Disease Research Laboratory (test for syphilis)
VSD	ventricular septal defect
VT	ventricular tachycardia
vWD	von Willebrand's disease
vWF	von Willebrand factor
VZIgG	varicella zoster immunoglobulin G
WAIS	Wechsler Adult Intelligence Scale
WCC	white cell count
WHO	World Health Organisation
WWII	World War II
ZIFT	zygote intrafallopian transfer

Part 1

EMQs and SBAs

Medicine

*Respiratory Medicine : Gastroenterology :
Nephrology : Cardiology : Connective Tissue
Disorders : Infectious Diseases : Skin Disorders :
Endocrine Disorders : Neurology : Haematology*

Chapter contributed by
Raja Dhar MBBS MRCP (UK) MD

Medicine EMQs

Theme: **Investigation of respiratory disease**

Options

A	CT PA	F	Scalene node biopsy
B	HRCT scanning	G	Skin-prick test
C	Lung volumes	H	Transfer factor
D	Mediastinoscopy	I	Ventilation–perfusion scan
E	Pleural biopsy	J	Walking distance of 6 minutes

Instructions

For each of the patients described below choose the SINGLE most appropriate investigation from the list of options above. Each option may be used once, more than once or not at all.

1 A 42-year-old man presents with sudden-onset severe shortness of breath and haemoptysis with an accompanying sharp drop in haemoglobin, which is out of proportion to the haemoptysis. His chest X-ray shows large areas of white-out in both lungs. ☐

2 A 45-year-old woman presents with a sudden-onset dry cough of 2 months' duration. She has painful, tender nodules in both shin areas. Her chest X-ray shows bilateral interstitial shadowing. ☐

3 A 66-year-old man with known lung cancer who is undergoing radiotherapy suddenly becomes acutely short of breath; he also has a sharp pain in the left side of his chest. Arterial blood measurement shows pH 7.38, $p(O_2)$ 8.6 kPa, $p(CO_2)$ 3.8 kPa and bicarbonate 22 mmol/l. ☐

4 A 68-year-old man presents complaining of a sudden-onset chest pain and gradually increasing shortness of breath over the last few months. Results of a chest X-ray requested by his GP show a large, right-sided pleural effusion. He worked as a lagger in a shipyard until the mid-1970s. ☐

5 A 32-year-old woman, an immigrant from Hong Kong, who was diagnosed with asthma when she was 18 years of age and has been treated for pneumonia on many occasions in the past, presents with gradually worsening breathlessness. Her chest X-rays demonstrate flitting pulmonary opacities. Results of a full blood count show Hb 14.2 g/dl, white cell count 13.8 × 10^9/l, differential count: lymphocytes 248 × 10^6/l, monocytes 138 × 10^6/l, neutrophils 1120 × 10^6/l, eosinophils 400 × 10^6/l.

Theme: **Management of obstructive airways diseases**

Options

A	Aminophylline tablets	G	N-acetylcysteine nebulisers
B	Combination of salmeterol and fluticasone	H	Pulmonary rehabilitation
		I	Salbutamol nebuliser
C	Fluticasone	J	Salmeterol
D	Ipratropium nebuliser	K	Tiotropium
E	Long-term oxygen therapy	L	Zafirlukast tablets
F	Magnesium sulphate		

Instructions

For each of the patients described below choose the SINGLE most appropriate agent from the list of options above. Each option may be used once, more than once or not at all.

6 A patient presents with severe COPD, an FEV_1 of 0.8 litres and three hospital admissions in the past year. Which evidence-based agent will reduce the acute exacerbation rates and improve quality of life with no impact on pulmonary function?

7 A patient with moderate COPD and an FEV_1 of 1.5 litres has been admitted to hospital twice this year (one admission last year). He is already on a salbutamol inhaler prn, an ipratropium inhaler four times a day and a combination of a steroid and a long-acting β-agonist. Which agent should be introduced after stopping one of his medications?

8 A 58-year-old man has severe COPD. Arterial blood gases on air when he was well showed pH 7.36, $p(O_2)$ 7.2 kPa and $p(CO_2)$ 6.6 kPa. An echocardiogram showed right ventricular dilatation and RV dysfunction. What is the only agent known to improve morbidity and mortality?

9 A 45-year-old woman with brittle asthma, using a salbutamol inhaler prn and a combination steroid and salmeterol inhaler, is experiencing acute flare-ups necessitating recurrent hospital admission. Which would be the next agent to introduce?   ☐

10 A 42-year-old woman with known asthma is on a salbutamol inhaler 200 μg prn and beclometasone 1000 μg bd. She has recurrent episodes of nocturnal awakening, cough and shortness of breath. Which would be the next agent to introduce?   ☐

11 A 26-year-old man has acute severe asthma. His peak flow was found to be 58% of predicted. He did not respond well to free-flow oxygen and the dose of oral steroid (prednisolone 40 mg) was repeated. Nebulisation was initially with salbutamol and then with a combination of salbutamol and ipratropium. Which agent should be used next?   ☐

Theme: **Pneumonia**

Options

A	Cytomegalovirus	E	*Pneumocystis jiroveci*
B	*Klebsiella pneumoniae*	F	*Pseudomonas aeruginosa*
C	*Legionella pneumophila*	G	Streptococcal pneumonia
D	*Mycoplasma pneumoniae*	H	Tuberculosis

Instructions

For each of the patients described below choose the SINGLE most appropriate answer from the list of options above. Each option may be used once, more than once or not at all.

12 A 56-year-old man with no underlying lung problems went on holiday to Cyprus. He developed a dry cough and cold, which seemed like a viral prodromal illness. After 4–5 days he felt confused and developed diarrhoea and vomiting. A blood test showed a white cell count of 116×10^9/l, neutrophils $10,100 \times 10^6$/l, lymphocytes 700×10^6/l, eosinophils 300×10^6/l, monocytes 500×10^6/l. He was also found to have hyponatraemia, hypoalbuminaemia and a high AST level. ☐

13 A 70-year-old woman with known COPD and diabetes presents with increased shortness of breath, some streaky haemoptysis and a cough that produces a purulent green sputum. Her chest X-ray revealed extensive bilateral consolidation. ☐

14 A 22-year-old man with known cystic fibrosis presents with a cough and breathlessness, which are much worse than usual. ☐

15 A 16-year-old boy living in an institution presents with headache and malaise that preceded chest symptoms by 48 hours. He has also developed a rash, predominantly on his arms and legs. Blood tests show a haemoglobin of 10.1 g/dl, a reticulocyte count of 5% and thrombocytopenia. His chest X-ray shows bilateral extensive shadowing in both lungs. ☐

16 A 58-year-old renal transplant recipient who is on ciclosporin
has developed a high fever, severe breathlessness and a dry
cough. His chest X-ray shows mild shadowing in the perihilar
region on the right side. Pulse oximetry demonstrates gross
desaturation on air.

Theme: **Diseases of the respiratory system**

Options

A	Ankylosing spondylitis	E	Goodpasture's syndrome
B	Churg–Strauss syndrome	F	Motor neurone disease
C	Cryptogenic organising pneumonia	G	Progressive massive fibrosis (PMF)
D	Extrinsic allergic alveolitis	H	Tropical pulmonary eosinophilia

Instructions

For each of the patients described below choose the SINGLE most appropriate answer from the list of options above. Each option may be used once, more than once or not at all.

17 A non-smoker who had worked in coal mines for 20 years presents with gradually increasing shortness of breath, limited exercise tolerance and a dry cough. His chest X-ray shows round fibrotic masses in the upper lobes with central cavitation. Lung function testing demonstrates a mixed restrictive and obstructive ventilatory defect with irreversible airflow limitation and reduced gas transfer. ☐

18 A 56-year-old man presents with breathlessness, which predominantly occurs when he is supine. He also has symptoms of sleep apnoea and daytime headaches and somnolence. Spirometry shows a decreased tidal volume and vital capacity. ☐

19 A 35-year-old man has been given a diagnosis of allergic rhinitis and asthma. Examination revealed a peripheral neuropathy with tingling and numbness in a 'glove and stocking' distribution. Skin lesions are present in the form of tender subcutaneous nodules. The patient is responding well to corticosteroids. ☐

20 A 48-year-old farmer presented with fever, malaise, cough and shortness of breath. On examination the patient was tachypnoeic, with coarse end-inspiratory crackles and wheeze throughout his chest. He was cyanosed. He also complained of severe weight loss. His chest X-ray shows fluffy nodular shadowing and there is a polymorphonuclear leucocytosis. ☐

Theme: **Lung cancer**

Options

A	Adenocarcinoma	E	Metastatic lung cancer
B	Alveolar-cell carcinoma	F	Pulmonary hamartoma
C	Bronchial carcinoid	G	Small-cell lung carcinoma
D	Large-cell carcinoma	H	Squamous-cell carcinoma

Instructions

For each of the statements given below choose the SINGLE most likely disease from the conditions listed above. Each option may be used once, more than once or not at all.

21 A lung cancer that presents with cavitation on chest X-ray, along with hypertrophic pulmonary osteoarthropathy. ☐

22 1–2% of lung tumours with a multicentric origin, sometimes associated with bronchorrhoea. ☐

23 This might arise from scar tissue, the pleura are commonly involved and it is associated with asbestos; more commonly seen than others. ☐

24 It arises from Kultchitsky cells, which are members of the APUD system and secrete polypeptide hormones. ☐

25 A slow-growing nodule seen on a CXR in the periphery of the lung; detected as an incidental finding on routine CXR. It has flecks of central calcification. ☐

26 A patient presented with recurrent haemoptysis. The CXR shows left lower lobe collapse. Bronchoscopy shows a cherry-red tumour. ☐

Theme: **Gastrointestinal bleeding**

Options

A Bacillary dysentery	G Irritable bowel syndrome
B Carcinoma of colon	H Ischaemic colitis
C Crohn's disease	I Mallory–Weiss syndrome
D Dieulafoy's gastric vascular	J Meckel's diverticulum
abnormality	K Portal gastropathy
E Diverticular disease	L Pseudoxanthoma elasticum
F Hereditary haemorrhagic	M Ulcerative colitis
telangiectasia	

Instructions

For each of the patients described below choose the SINGLE most likely diagnosis from the list of options above. Each option may be used once, more than once or not at all.

27 A 54-year-old man presents with diarrhoea containing blood and mucus, urgency and tenesmus. He has aphthous ulceration in his mouth. ☐   M

28 An 82-year-old, hypertensive woman presents with sudden-onset abdominal pain and passage of bright-red blood per rectum but with little diarrhoea. On examination her abdomen is distended and tender. Rigid sigmoidoscopy shows a normal mucosal appearance with some blood. ☐   H

29 A 79-year-old woman underwent bifemoral aortic surgery (prosthesis) 25 days ago. She was re-admitted to hospital with haematemesis and melaena and evidence of haemodynamic compromise. An emergency endoscopy was performed after a series of ice-cold gastric lavage. The source of bleeding has now become visible after successful aspiration of blood and good manoeuvring. ☐

30 A 24-year-old woman has been admitted for investigation of recurrent GI bleeding. Further examination reveals a papular rash, retinal angioid streaks and stenosis of the cardiac coronary artery. Upper gastrointestinal endoscopy reveals vascular dilatation in the gastric body. ☐

31 A 28-year-old man attends A&E with haematemesis after an active bout of drinking over the weekend. He has a history of repeated bouts of retching after drinking. ☐

Theme: **Malabsorption**

Options

A   Bacterial overgrowth   E   Intestinal resection
B   Coeliac disease   F   Radiation enteritis
C   Dermatitis herpetiformis   G   Tropical sprue
D   *Giardia* infestation   H   Whipple's disease

Instructions

For each of the patients described below choose the SINGLE most likely diagnosis from the list of options above. Each option may be used once, more than once or not at all.

32 A 45-year-old woman presents with tiredness and malaise associated with anaemia; she also has symptoms of diarrhoea and steatorrhoea. Her history shows that she was infertile and suffered from anxiety and depression. She also has osteoporosis. ☐

33 A 44-year-old woman on long-term antibiotics for recurrent UTI gives a history of steatorrhoea and diarrhoea of 3 months' duration. She is found to be vitamin B_{12} deficient. ☐

34 A 38-year-old man presents with a painful abdomen and steatorrhoea, along with significant weight loss. He also has cervical lymphadenopathy and small-joint arthropathy. ☐

35 A 40-year-old businessman recently returned from India presents with diarrhoea, malabsorption and steatorrhoea. ☐

Theme: **Diseases of the small intestine**

Options

A	Abetalipoproteinaemia	F	Meckel's diverticulum
B	Amyloidosis	G	Protein-losing enteropathy
C	Eosinophilic gastroenteritis	H	Small intestinal ischaemia
D	Gastroenteritis	I	Systemic sclerosis
E	Intestinal lymphangiectasia	J	Tuberculosis

Instructions

For each of the patients described below choose the SINGLE most likely diagnosis from the list of options above. Each option may be used once, more than once or not at all.

36 A patient with steatorrhoea has been found to have a low serum immunoglobulin level, a low number of circulating lymphocytes and hypoproteinaemia with ankle oedema.

37 A patient with diarrhoea and steatorrhoea has spiky red blood cells on a peripheral blood film, mental retardation and peripheral neuropathy.

38 An African immigrant with fever, anorexia and weight loss presents acutely with intestinal obstruction. On examination there is a palpable lump in his right iliac fossa.

39 A 28-year-old man with a history of asthma presented with abdominal pain, nausea and vomiting. On examination he was found to have high blood and tissue IgE levels. He responded well to steroids.

40 A 68-year-old man presents with hypertension and recurrent bouts of abdominal pain that occur after the ingestion of food. Auscultation of his abdomen reveals loud bruits.

Theme: **Colonic disorders**

Options

A	Crohn's disease	E	Ischaemic colitis
B	Diverticulitis	F	Megacolon
C	Functional diarrhoea	G	Pneumatosis cystoides intestinalis
D	Irritable bowel syndrome	H	Ulcerative colitis

Instructions

For each of the results described below choose the SINGLE most likely diagnosis from the list of options above. Each option may be used once, more than once or not at all.

41 Barium follow-through in this condition reveals asymmetrical alteration in the mucosal pattern. The findings may vary from mild, patchy, superficial ulceration to more widespread larger and deeper ulcers.

A

42 Plain abdominal X-ray with abdominal ultrasound are the key investigations for this disease. The extent of disease can be judged by the distribution of air in the colon and the presence of colonic dilatation. An unprepared barium enema would show superficial ulceration and a shortened and narrow colon in patients with long-standing disease.

F

43 A full-thickness colonic biopsy is diagnostic in this condition. A frozen section is stained for acetylcholinesterase. Manometric studies will show failure of relaxation of the internal sphincter.

F

44 A spiral CT of the lower abdomen in this condition would show colonic wall thickening and pericolic collections. Increased density extending into the immediate pericolic fat with thickening of the pelvic fascial planes would also been seen.

B

45 Patients with this condition, who often have COPD, are diagnosed on the basis of radiography of the abdomen, a barium enema or sigmoidoscopy.

G

Theme: **Diarrhoea**

Options

A Behçet's disease	G Paget's disease
B *Campylobacter* diarrhoea	H Pseudomembranous
C Carcinoid syndrome	enterocolitis
D Fungal diarrhoea	I Purgative abuse
E Irritable bowel syndrome	J Thyrotoxicosis
F Medullary carcinoma of the	K Zollinger–Ellison syndrome
thyroid	

Instructions

For each of the patients described below choose the SINGLE most likely diagnosis from the list of options above. Each option may be used once, more than once or not at all.

46 A 36-year-old woman presented with large-volume diarrhoea (more than 1 litre/day). Sigmoidoscopy shows a pigmented mucosa and a rectal biopsy shows the presence of pigment-laden macrophages.

47 A 36-year-old man of Japanese descent presented with recurrent oral ulceration and anterior uveitis. Over a short period he has become confused and has developed diarrhoea, abdominal pain and loss of appetite.

48 A previously fit 22-year-old man presented with acute bloody diarrhoea, crampy abdominal pain and low-grade fever. The symptoms resolved spontaneously in 6 days and have not recurred.

49 A 26-year-old sales manager presented with a 4-month history of diarrhoea alternating with constipation. He is known to suffer from hyperventilation states. His stools were soft and there was no history of vomiting or bleeding. No abnormality was found on examination. All investigations, including flexible fibreoptic sigmoidoscopy and radiography are normal.

50 A 45-year-old man presents with diarrhoea and dysphagia. He also complains that his voice has changed during the last 2 weeks.

Theme: **Diagnosis of connective tissue disorders**

Options

A   Antiphospholipid antibody
    syndrome
B   Limited cutaneous
    scleroderma
C   Overlap syndrome

D   Polymyalgia rheumatica
E   Polymyositis
F   Rheumatoid arthritis
G   Sjögren's syndrome
H   Systemic lupus erythematosus

Instructions

*For each of the patients described below choose the SINGLE most likely
diagnosis from the list of options above. Each option may be used once,
more than once or not at all.*

51 A 32-year-old woman has raised ESR and CPK levels, as well as
small rises in transaminase and aldolase levels. EMG shows a
spontaneous fibrillation potential and salvos of repetitive
potentials. ☐

52 A 42-year-old man has normocytic normochromic anaemia and
is positive for rheumatoid factor. X-ray of his hands shows
deposits of calcium around his fingers. A barium swallow
demonstrates impaired oesophageal motility. Urine microscopy
shows proteinuria and he has reduced creatinine clearance. ☐

53 A 42-year-old woman is found to have pancytopenia, positive
rheumatoid factor, reduced complement levels and a positive
VDRL. CT scan of her brain showed an infarct and evidence of
premature cerebral atrophy. ☐

54 A 45-year-old man has raised immunoglobulin levels, positive
rheumatoid factor, positive antinuclear antibody. He also has
filamentary keratitis, which was shown up on Rose Bengal
staining of his eyes. ☐

Theme: **Presentation of autoimmune diseases**

Options

A	Antiphospholipid antibody syndrome	E	Polymyositis
B	Hashimoto's thyroiditis	F	Rheumatoid arthritis
C	Overlap syndrome	G	Sjögren's syndrome
D	Pernicious anaemia	H	Systemic lupus erythematosus
		I	Systemic sclerosis

Instructions

For each of the patients described below choose the SINGLE most likely diagnosis from the list of options above. Each option may be used once, more than once or not at all.

55 A 45-year-old woman presents acutely with atrial fibrillation. She has pain in her small joints (which, however, look clinically normal) and photosensitive palmar-plantar rashes. Dipstick urinalysis shows large amounts of protein. ☐

56 A 32-year-old woman presents with dyspareunia, non-progressive polyarthritis and long-standing polyuria, which had been diagnosed in the past as nephrogenic diabetes insipidus. She is also on medication for depression. ☐

57 A 45-year-old woman has a history of two past episodes of TIA and epilepsy. She is also known to have aortic regurgitation. A full blood count reveals thrombocytopenia. ☐

58 A 45-year-old man with deforming small-joint arthritis is found to have bilateral interstitial shadowing on a chest X-ray. Further examination reveals nail-fold infarcts. ☐

Theme: **Inflammatory arthritis**

Options

A	Ankylosing spondylitis	E	Palindromic rheumatism
B	Enteropathic arthritis	F	Psoriatic arthropathy
C	Gout	G	Reactive arthritis
D	Lyme's arthritis	H	Rheumatoid arthritis

Instructions

For each of the patients described below choose the SINGLE most likely diagnosis from the list of options above. Each option may be used once, more than once or not at all.

59 A 22-year-old man presents with backache, pain in his right hip and a fixed flexion deformity. There is a history of recurrent redness of the eyes. His mother had a similar problem, although it was of a milder intensity. ☐

60 A 34-year-old woman presents with limited small-joint arthritis. The joints are deformed and unsightly but have good functional ability. In addition, there is associated nail dystrophy. X-rays show central erosions in the joints.   *Psoriasis*   ☐

61 A 40-year-old man presents with acute, asymmetrical, lower limb arthritis following a viral chest infection. He says he has difficulty walking due to the pain. Further examination reveals nail dystrophy and bilateral redness of the eyes. ☐

62 A 52-year-old man with known heart failure and on treatment developed an agonising pain and swelling of his right thumb. The pain and swelling has now subsided with treatment, after about 72 hours. ☐

63 On his return some years ago from a visit to New Jersey, USA, this man developed a large reddish rash, later followed by multiple rashes in close proximity. He then suffered chills and fever. Although the symptoms gradually subsided within a few weeks, for many years he has been left with swelling and pain in his large joints. ☐

Theme: **Imaging techniques for renal diseases**

Options

A	Antegrade pyelography	G	Renal arteriography
B	CT scan	H	Renal biopsy
C	Excretion urography	I	Renal scintigraphy
D	Micturating cystography	J	Retrograde pyelography
E	MRI	K	USS
F	Plain X-ray		

Instructions

For each of the investigations described below choose the SINGLE most likely diagnosis from the list of options above. Each option may be used once, more than once or not at all.

64 This investigation provides functional evidence of obstruction. It may also be carried out before and after the administration of an ACE inhibitor to diagnose functional arterial stenosis. ☐

65 This is carried out in patients with recurrent UTI, especially in adults with disturbed bladder function, when it can be combined with urodynamic measurements of bladder pressure and urethral flow. ☐

66 It is increasingly being used as a first-line investigation in patients with suspected ureteric colic. This investigation is also used to evaluate the retroperitoneum for tumours and retroperitoneal fibrosis and other causes of ureteric obstruction. ☐

67 This is the investigation of choice for carrying out renal measurements, diagnosing polycystic kidney disease and detecting renal vein thrombosis. ☐

Theme: **Diagnosis of renal diseases**

Options

A	Acute tubulointerstitial nephritis	E	Haemolytic uraemic syndrome
B	Analgesic nephropathy	F	Medullary cystic kidney disease
C	Balkan nephropathy	G	Retroperitoneal fibrosis
D	Contrast nephropathy	H	Thrombotic thrombocytopenic purpura

Instructions

For each of the patients described below choose the SINGLE most likely diagnosis from the list of options above. Each option may be used once, more than once or not at all.

68 A 24-year-old body-builder presented with a cellulitis of his left arm. He was started on oral penicillin V by his GP. After the second dose he has now developed fever, arthralgia, a skin rash and acute oliguric renal failure. ☐

69 A 30-year-old woman suffered a bout of gastroenteritis, followed by rapidly rising urea and creatinine levels. A full blood count shows thrombocytopenia. ☐

70 A 16-year-old girl developed polyuria, polydipsia and growth retardation. There is a family history of a similar problem. A renal biopsy clinches the diagnosis. ☐

71 A 62-year-old man with a previous history of surgery for abdominal aortic aneurysm, presented with malaise, backache and normochromic anaemia, uraemia and a raised ESR. A periaortic mass is seen on CT scanning. ☐

Theme: **Management of renal failure**

Options

A	Antihypertensives	G	Haemofiltration
B	Calcium gluconate	H	Insulin + dextrose
C	Calcium resonium	I	Intravenous fluid
D	CAPD	J	Intravenous furosemide
E	Catheterisation	K	Oral phosphodiesterase
F	Haemodialysis		inhibitor

Instructions

For each of the patients described below choose the SINGLE most likely management from the list of options above. Each option may be used once, more than once or not at all.

72 A 65-year-old man receiving CAPD for hypertensive nephropathy complains of distressing impotence. There is no history of coronary artery disease.

73 A 64-year-old man with end-stage renal disease, severe coronary artery disease and limited exercise tolerance due to COPD, and a colostomy due to a past history of ulcerative colitis, suffers acute deterioration in his renal status.

74 An 85-year-old man presents with anuria for the past 72 hours. He is confused and restless. Examination reveals a distended lower abdomen. Examination of his chest reveals features consistent with pulmonary oedema and a small right-sided pleural effusion. His potassium level is 5.8 mmol/l, urea 40 mmol/l and creatinine 760 μmol/l.

75 A 42-year-old, previously healthy, man presents with a traumatic fracture of the neck of femur. A large haematoma is drained during the surgery. Since the operation he has had a few bouts of vomiting and complains of thirst and malaise. His sodium level is 152 mmol/l, potassium 3.4 mmol/l, urea 26 mmol/l and creatinine 176 μmol/l.

76 A 62-year-old man with a CABG is taking furosemide, perindropril and spironolactone for heart failure. His potassium level has persistently been between 6.0 mmol/l and 6.5 mmol/l for the past 3 months. He is asymptomatic with no ECG changes. ☐

Theme: **Treatment of cardiac arrhythmias**

Options

A	Amiodarone	E	Flecainide
B	Cardiac pacemaker	F	Intravenous adenosine
C	Carotid sinus massage	G	Metoprolol
D	Disopyramide	H	Verapamil

Instructions

For each of the patients described below choose the SINGLE most likely management from the list of options above. Each option may be used once, more than once or not at all.

77 A 66-year-old man with a previous history of IHD, and a past CABG, presents to the hospital after a brief episode of angina. Further questioning reveals that he experiences intermittent angina attacks. ECG shows AF at 140 bpm. ☐

78 A 56-year-old man with a previous history of palpitations presents to the hospital with a history of syncope. A 24-h tape recording shows multiple 4-s to 6-s sinus pauses, interspersed with episodes of paroxysmal atrial tachyarrhythmias at a rate of up to 180 bpm. ☐

79 A 24-year-old man presents to the hospital on a Monday after a weekend of binge-drinking in Blackpool. He is found to have AF at 150 bpm. Echo shows normal underlying cardiac function. There is no other co-morbidity. ☐

80 A 56-year-old woman with no history of IHD presents with syncope. In hospital she had a sustained episode of ventricular tachycardia with a blood pressure of 110/60 mmHg. She complains of palpitations, but no dizziness, during this episode. ☐

Theme: **Results of cardiac investigations**

Options

A	Atrial myxoma	F	Mitral valve prolapse
B	Atrial septal defect	G	PDA
C	Constrictive pericarditis	H	Prosthetic heart valve endocarditis
D	HOCM	I	Vasovagal syncope
E	IHD	J	VSD

Instructions

For each of the results of the investigations described below choose the SINGLE most likely diagnosis from the list of options above. Each option may be used once, more than once or not at all.

81 Echo shows small ventricular cavities, normal wall thickness and dilated atria. Cardiac catheterisation shows pressure equalisation in all four chambers. ☐

82 ECG shows some degree of RBBB. Echo shows RV hypertrophy and pulmonary artery dilatation, and abnormal motion of the IVS. ☐

83 Echo shows posterior movement of one or both mitral valve cusps into the left atrium during systole. ☐

84 Echo shows more hypertrophy of the septum of the left ventricle than the posterior wall, systolic forward motion of the mitral valve and a vigorously contracting ventricle. Exercise testing and ambulatory ECG monitoring provide prognostic information. ☐

85 Echo shows a small space-occupying lesion in the left atrium. ☐

Theme: **Viral illness**

Options

A	Arenavirus	F	Human herpesvirus 8
B	Coxsackievirus	G	Poliovirus
C	Cytomegalovirus	H	Rubella virus
D	Ebola virus disease	I	Yellow fever virus
E	Epstein–Barr virus		

Instructions

For each of the patients described below choose the SINGLE most likely virus from the list of options above. Each option may be used once, more than once or not at all.

86 A 56-year-old woman returned from an African safari with a high fever, headache, a flushed face and conjunctival suffusion. There was some epigastric pain and vomiting. Examination revealed a relative bradycardia. Her fever subsided, but it has now returned and with deepening jaundice and hepatomegaly. She is bleeding from her gums and vomiting, and the vomitus has a 'coffee-ground' appearance. ☐

87 A 16-year-old adolescent presents complaining of a mild conjunctivitis and lymphadenopathy that has been followed by the appearance of a rash on her forehead, which has gone on to involve her trunk and limbs. It is macular and discrete. She has mild splenomegaly. She describes having had some petechial lesions on her soft palate. ☐

88 A 22-year-old man with a history of a recent tonsillectomy initially presented with fever and myalgia. These symptoms have persisted for some days, but he has now developed progressive paraparesis. He has also developed difficulty in swallowing, aspiration and a nasal intonation of his voice. ☐

89 A 19-year-old man initially presented with fever, headache and a sore throat. Cervical lymph nodes were palpable, especially the posterior cervical lymph nodes. There was a mild splenomegaly. He gradually recovered but has remained depressed for several months after the episode. ☐

Theme: **Bacterial illness**

Options

A	Actinomycosis	F	Nocardiasis
B	Anthrax	G	Plague
C	Leprosy	H	Q fever
D	Leptospirosis	I	Tularaemia
E	Listeriosis		

Instructions

For each of the patients described below choose the SINGLE most likely diagnosis from the list of options above. Each option may be used once, more than once or not at all.

90 A 26-year-old man presented with high fever, chill, headache and vomiting, followed by severe prostration. This was followed by the development of lymphadenopathy in the inguinal region. Within a period of 7 days sinuses had formed, with the discharge of pus. ☐

91 A 36-year-old woman developed a small, erythematous maculopapular rash on her arm: initially, this was painless. It later evolved into a vesicle that has now ulcerated, with the formation of a central black eschar. Axillary lymph nodes on the same side are enlarged. ☐

92 A 28-year-old Egyptian man presented with a skin rash in the form of macules, papules, nodules and plaques in different stages of evolution. The involvement was most noticeable on the earlobes. There was peripheral oedema and rhinitis. He has gone on to develop glove-and-stocking anaesthesia and gynaecomastia. ☐

93 A 32-year-old woman on a holiday to Hawaii developed a severe headache, malaise and myalgia. There was conjunctival suffusion. Examination revealed hepatosplenomegaly, lymphadenopathy and skin rash. Following the initial symptoms the patient has developed jaundice, renal failure and a haemolytic anaemia. ☐

Theme: **Fungal and protozoal illnesses**

Options

A	Amoebiasis	F	Giardiasis
B	Aspergillosis	G	Histoplasmosis
C	Chagas' disease	H	Leishmaniasis
D	Coccidioidomycosis	I	Malaria
E	Cryptosporidiosis	J	*Pneumocystis jiroveci* infection

(handwritten annotation: Benznidazole near Chagas' disease; Quinine near Malaria)

Instructions

For each of the patients described below choose the SINGLE most likely disease from the list of options above. Each option may be used once, more than once or not at all.

94 A 32-year-old man on a visit to Mexico developed a fever, malaise, cough and expectoration. This was followed by erythema nodosum on both shins and phlyctenular conjunctivitis. Chest X-ray revealed multiple cavities. Diagnosis has been made on the basis of serological tests. ☐

95 A 24-year-old immigrant returned to India to visit his family. He developed fever with malaise, headache and vomiting. He continued to deteriorate rapidly, with oliguria. Blood examination revealed anaemia and features consistent with DIC. He has become stuporous and confused and has developed convulsions. ☐

96 A 32-year-old man from Uganda had short-lasting episodes of fever and lymphadenopathy which occurred over a period of years. Examination revealed hepatosplenomegaly. After about 5 years the patient developed persistent headache and some behavioural changes, with confusion and daytime somnolence. The disease progressed and he has now developed tremor and ataxia. ☐

97 A 26-year-old man, just back from the tropics, developed watery diarrhoea, nausea, anorexia and abdominal bloating. His stool became pale, in spite of treatment, with features suggestive of steatorrhoea. This has now been followed by weight loss. ☐

Theme: **Chronic immunodeficiency syndromes**

Options

A	Ataxia telangiectasia	F	IgA deficiency
B	Chédiak–Higashi syndrome	G	Severe combined
C	Chronic granulomatous disease ×2 R		immunodeficiency
D	Combined variable	H	Wiskott–Aldrich syndrome
	immunodeficiency	I	X-linked
E	DiGeorge syndrome		hypogammaglobulinaemia

Instructions

For each of the patients described below choose the SINGLE most likely diagnosis from the list of options above. Each option may be used once, more than once or not at all.

98 A 16-year-old boy presented with chronic suppurative abscesses affecting his skin. There was generalised lymphadenopathy. Screening revealed abscesses in his lungs and his liver. He has experienced recurrent chest infections and colonisation by opportunistic infections like atypical *Mycobacteria, Nocardia* and *Salmonella* spp. Diagnosis has been made by the nitroblue tetrazolium test. ☐

99 This child presented with mucocutaneous candidiasis and diarrhoea. The patient has dysmorphic facies. Auscultation of the heart has revealed a ventricular septal defect. He is also hypocalcaemic. VSD ↓ Ca ☐

100 This child presented with eczema and thrombocytopenia. Later on, he developed Hodgkin's disease. An underlying defect is found to be X-linked. ☐

101 This child presented in the third week of life with a failure to thrive and severe bacterial infections. Tests have revealed lymphopenia and hypogammaglobulinaemia. Even with supportive and antimicrobial therapy the patient has a very poor prognosis. ☐

Theme: **Vitamin deficiency**

Options

A	Niacin	E	Vitamin B_6
B	Riboflavin	F	Vitamin C
C	Vitamin A	G	Vitamin E
D	Vitamin B_1	H	Vitamin K

Instructions

For each of the patients described below choose the SINGLE most likely deficiency from the list of options above. Each option may be used once, more than once or not at all.

102 A 26-year-old Asian man presented to his GP with bleeding gums and spontaneous bruising. Examination revealed swollen, spongy gums with superadded infection and perifollicular haemorrhage. A blood test shows this man to be anaemic.

103 A man of African descent presents to his GP complaining of chronic diarrhoea and recurrent mouth ulcers. He is chronically depressed and tired. He has photodermatitis on the sun-exposed parts of his body, together with redness, cracks and occasional ulceration.

104 A 62-year-old man of Vietnamese descent presented with heaviness and stiffness in his legs, followed by numbness and pins-and-needles sensations. The ankle jerk was absent. He has developed florid signs of polyneuropathy involving his arms and legs, as well as ataxia, cognitive deficit, nystagmus and bilateral rectus palsy.

105 A 72-year-old man, with a prolonged recovery from surgery for an abdominal aortic aneurysm, presents with angular stomatitis, a red inflamed tongue, seborrhoeic dermatitis involving his face (especially around his nose) and scrotum, and conjunctivitis with vascularisation of the cornea.

Theme: **Skin disorders**

Options

A	Atopic eczema	E	Pityriasis rosea
B	Granuloma annulare	F	Seborrhoeic eczema
C	Guttate psoriasis	G	Urticaria
D	Lichen planus		

Instructions

For each of the patients described below choose the SINGLE most likely diagnosis from the list of options above. Each option may be used once, more than once or not at all.

106 A 56-year-old man receiving gold therapy for known rheumatoid arthritis has developed an intensely pruritic rash on his lower legs. The rash appears as purple, flat-topped polygonal papules surmounted by a white pattern. Oral and anogenital involvement is present. ☐

107 A 26-year-old prisoner recovering from a chest infection developed a pink-coloured, scaly rash over his trunk. The lesions followed the dermatomal lines. They were asymptomatic. These have now spontaneously resolved after 6 weeks. ☐

108 A 26-year-old man was recovering from a streptococcal sore throat. He was found to have raindrop-like lesions over his trunk, which have resolved spontaneously over 6 weeks without treatment. ☐

109 A 25-year-old diabetic woman developed a papular rash on the dorsum of her hands and feet. The rash was flesh-coloured, with an erythematous margin. A skin biopsy showed a granulomatous dermal infiltrate. She is being treated with cryotherapy. ☐

Theme: **Treatment for parkinsonism**

Options

A	Amantidine	F	Co-beneldopa (Madopar®)
B	Apomorphine		containing levodopa + benserazide
C	Benzatropine	G	Lisuride
D	Bromocriptine *OA* *agonist*	H	Ropinirole *OA agonist*
E	Levodopa	I	Stereotactic surgery

Instructions

For each of the patients described below choose the SINGLE most likely treatment from the list of options above. Each option may be used once, more than once or not at all.

110 A 62-year-old man was prescribed a tricyclic antidepressant by his GP. Although the symptoms of depression have improved, he has gradually slowed down and developed rigidity, with recurrent episodes of falling. ☐

111 A 52-year-old man with known parkinsonism has been on levodopa therapy for a few years. He has now started to develop dyskinesias a few hours after taking his medication and reports having episodes when he is frozen in space. ☐

112 A patient with Parkinson's disease was tried on different drugs but with gradual waning of response. She has now developed severe rigidity, akinesis and drooling of saliva and has difficulty in swallowing. ☐

113 A 70-year-old man developed symptoms that were thought to be related to idiopathic parkinsonism. These limited his activities of daily life. The combination of levodopa and carbidopa did not smooth out the 'on and off' effects. He has since been changed over to another agent, with good response. ☐

Theme: **Investigations for CNS disorders**

Options

A	Cataplexy	F	Huntington's disease
B	Cerebral abscess	G	Multiple sclerosis
C	Duchenne's muscle dystrophy	H	Myasthenia gravis
D	Friedreich's ataxia	I	Narcolepsy
E	Guillain–Barré syndrome	J	Syringomyelia

Instructions

For each of the statements described below choose the SINGLE most likely diagnosis from the list of options above. Each option may be used once, more than once or not at all.

114 Nerve conduction-velocity studies in this condition show slowing of conduction, prolonged distal motor latency with or without conduction block. ☐

115 CSF protein is typically elevated in this condition. The cell count and sugar level remain normal. MRI may be diagnostic. CSF examination will show immunoglobulin production within the CNS in response to antigen, and a raised mononuclear cell count of 5–60 cells/mm³. ☐

116 This condition is strongly associated with HLA-DR2 and HLA-DQB1 0602 antigens. Patients also have subnormal hypocretin-1 levels in their CSF. ☐

117 A combination of disease-specific IgG antibodies and a decrement of evoked muscle action potentials following continued stimulation of motor nerves helps to clinch the diagnosis. ☐

Theme: **CNS disorders**

Options

A   Cortical venous thrombosis
B   Creutzfeldt–Jakob disease
C   Huntington's disease
D   Idiopathic intracranial hypertension

E   Normal-pressure hydrocephalus
F   Subacute sclerosing panencephalitis
G   Syringomyelia   pain + temp ↓
H   Tabes dorsalis

Instructions

For each of the patients described below choose the SINGLE most likely diagnosis from the list of options above. Each option may be used once, more than once or not at all.

118 A 26-year-old man presents with pain in an upper limb, which is aggravated by coughing. He has difficulty in walking due to weakness in his legs and has muscle wasting in his hands and the forearm.   ☐

119 A 36-year-old overweight woman, with a history of menstrual irregularities, complains of recurrent headaches and visual blurring. Examination reveals a right-sided VIth nerve palsy. There is severe papilloedema.   ☐

120 A 32-year-old man was found to have neuropsychiatric problems. This was followed by the development of ataxia and dementia with myoclonus or chorea.   ☐

121 A 36-year-old man developed lightning pains in his trunk and both arms and this was followed by the development of ataxia and a stamping gait. Examination reveals muscle wasting in both upper and lower limbs and sensory loss. There is ptosis and optic atrophy.   Argyll   ☐

122 A 42-year-old man with a positive family history developed abnormal limb movements and presenile dementia. Treatment is with phenothiazines, with an aim to cause parkinsonism. Tetrabenazine has helped to control movements.   ☐

123 A 46-year-old woman with a previous history of sinusitis developed headache, a raised temperature and chemosis of the conjunctiva. A lumbar puncture showed raised intracranial pressure, but no other sign of meningitis. Within the next 24 hours she developed a left-sided VIth nerve palsy and right-sided VIth and IIIrd nerve palsies. MRI has revealed the diagnosis.

Theme: **Typical stroke syndromes**

Options

A   Anton's disease
B   Binswanger's disease
C   Lateral medullary syndrome
D   Locked-in syndrome
E   Parinaud's disease

F   Persistent vegetative state
G   Pseudobulbar palsy
H   Watershed cerebral infarction
I   Weber's syndrome

Instructions

For each of the patients described below choose the SINGLE most likely diagnosis from the list of options above. Each option may be used once, more than once or not at all.

124 A 62-year-old man presented to the hospital complaining of facial numbness, diplopia and difficulty in maintaining his balance. Examination reveals nystagmus, ataxia, Horner's syndrome and IXth and Xth cranial nerve palsies. ☐

125 A man has a history of multiple TIAs, dementia and hypertension. A CT scan shows low-attenuation regions in the cerebral white matter. ☐

126 A 72-year-old man who presented with stroke, has been found to have a IIIrd nerve paralysis and contralateral hemiplegia. There is paralysis of upward gaze. ☐

127 An 80-year-old man is in a state of unresponsiveness. He is fully aware but unable to communicate except by vertical eye movements. ☐

intact spinothalamic
damaged medial lemniscus
basilar artery damage

Theme: **Endocrine diseases**

Options

A	Conn's syndrome	E	Hashimoto's thyroiditis
B	Cushing's disease	F	Medullary carcinoma of the
C	De-Quervain's thyroiditis		thyroid
D	Ectopic ACTH-producing	G	Nelson's syndrome
	tumour	H	Phaeochromocytoma

Instructions

For each of the patients described below choose the SINGLE most likely diagnosis from the list of options above. Each option may be used once, more than once or not at all.

128 A 32-year-old woman presented with fever, malaise, pain in her neck, and tachycardia. Examination reveals tremor and tenderness in her neck. The ESR is raised. ☐

129 A 74-year-old smoker presented to his GP with cough and shortness of breath. Examination reveals pigmentation of the oral mucosa and also over his palms and soles. Tests show he is diabetic and hypokalaemic. ☐

130 A 45-year-old man presented to his GP with vague symptoms of headache, proximal muscle weakness and nocturia. Test results show him to be severely hypertensive (230/130 mmHg) and hypokalaemic. ☐

131 A 32-year-old diabetic man has repeatedly been admitted to hospital for what was described as anxiety or panic attacks and palpitations. On this occasion he is found to be tremulous and hypertensive. A persistent weight loss is noted. There are no other features of note. ☐

Theme: **Overdoses**

Options

A	Amphetamines	E	Cocaine
B	Aspirin	F	Organophosphate insecticides
C	Cannabis	G	Theophylline
D	Carbon monoxide	H	Tricyclic antidepressants

Instructions

For each of the patients described below choose the SINGLE most likely agent from the list of options above. Each option may be used once, more than once or not at all.

132 A 26-year-old man changed his job from a labourer to a paint stripper. About 2 months into his new job he went to his GP complaining of recurrent bouts of headaches and mild exertional dyspnoea. The GP diagnosed a viral illness. However, the symptoms did not go away and during the next 2 months his symptoms gradually became worse. He was brought to hospital with generalised tonic-clonic convulsions, which was followed by a cardiorespiratory arrest. ☐

133 A 66-year-old man with known asthma was brought to hospital with nausea and vomiting and a single episode of haematemesis. He also complained of central abdominal pain and diarrhoea. His ECG shows supraventricular tachycardia at 150 bpm. Blood tests show hypokalaemia and acidaemia. ☐

134 A 56-year-old farmer was brought into hospital with nausea, vomiting, abdominal colic and diarrhoea. He also complained of chest tightness. Examination of the eyes revealed miosis. Diagnosis has been confirmed by measuring erythrocyte acetylcholinesterase activity. ☐

135 A 26-year-old woman presented with hyperventilation, sweating, nausea, vomiting and epigastric pain. Blood gas analysis shows a mixed acid-base disturbance with respiratory alkalosis and metabolic acidosis. ☐

Theme: **Common adverse effects of drugs in pregnancy**

Options

A	Damage to bone and teeth	D	Neonatal goitre
B	Hare lip, cleft palate and cardiac abnormality ✓↳	E	Neural tube defect
		F	Renal damage and oligohydramnios
C	Methaemoglobinaemia and haemolysis in neonates	G	Vestibular damage

Instructions

For each of the patients described below choose the SINGLE most likely abnormality attributable to their treatment from the list of options above. Each option may be used once, more than once or not at all.

136 A 32-year-old Asian immigrant who is 30 weeks' pregnant developed fever with shaking chills and rigor. She was diagnosed with malaria and prescribed chloroquine. ☐

137 A 30-year-old woman who was 18 weeks' pregnant was given a diagnosis of trigeminal neuralgia and prescribed carbamazepine. ☐

138 A 26-year-old woman who presented to A&E with a second fit was prescribed phenytoin as anticonvulsant medication. ☐

139 A 28-year-old woman was prescribed tetracycline at 34 weeks' gestation for recurrent UTIs. ☐

Theme: **Haematological malignancies**

Options

A	Acute lymphoblastic leukaemia	F	Hodgkin's disease
B	Acute myelogenous leukaemia	G	Myeloma
C	Burkitt's lymphoma	H	Non-Hodgkin's lymphoma
D	Chronic lymphoblastic leukaemia	I	Prolymphocytic leukaemia
E	Hairy-cell leukaemia	J	Waldenström's macroglobulinaemia

Instructions

For each of the patients described below choose the SINGLE most likely diagnosis from the list of options above. Each option may be used once, more than once or not at all.

140 A 64-year-old man was investigated for recurrent chest infections. Tests show he has haemolytic anaemia and a positive Coombs' test. His platelet count is normal. Examination reveals the presence of a few enlarged peripheral lymph nodes and splenomegaly. ☐

141 A 56-year-old man is in bone marrow failure, with anaemia, thrombocytopenia and neutropenia. He has undergone splenectomy for an enlarged spleen and is receiving fludarabine. ☐

142 A 36-year-old man presented with fever, night sweats and weight loss. Examination shows hepatosplenomegaly and cervical lymph node enlargement. Cell counts are normal but with a raised ESR. CXR shows mediastinal widening. A bone marrow film shows clonal B-lymphocyte proliferation. ☐

143 An 18-year-old man from Uganda presented with a jaw tumour. Examination reveals hepatomegaly. Antibodies to the Epstein–Barr virus are present in his serum. ☐

144 A 66-year-old man presented with sudden-onset severe backache and was thought to have vertebral collapse with hypercalcaemia. Blood examination shows anaemia, neutropenia and thrombocytopenia. There is associated renal impairment. □

145 A 76-year-old man presented with headache and visual disturbance, generalised malaise and weight loss. His ESR is raised and a bone marrow film reveals lymphoplasmacytoid cells. Protein electrophoresis demonstrates the presence of IgM paraprotein. □

Theme: **Coagulation disorders**

Options

A   Antiphospholipid antibody
    syndrome
B   Disseminated intravascular
    coagulation
C   Excessive fibrinolysis

D   Haemophilia A
E   Haemophilia B
F   Liver disease
G   Vitamin K deficiency
H   von Willebrand's disease

Instructions

*For each of the patients described below choose the SINGLE most likely
diagnosis from the list of options above. Each option may be used once,
more than once or not at all.*

146 A 16-year-old adolescent undergoing an appendicectomy was
found to bleed unusually during and after the surgery. Routine
coagulation tests show a prolonged APTT but his PT and
bleeding time are normal.

147 A 24-year-old woman presented with menorrhagia to her GP.
A routine coagulation test shows a normal PT, prolonged
APTT and prolonged bleeding time.

148 A malnourished child from Ghana was taken to his GP with
recurrent episodes of epistaxis. Coagulation tests show a
prolonged PT and APTT, with a normal bleeding time.

149 A 36-year-old pregnant woman developed a UTI. Urine
culture revealed Gram-negative rods. She developed a high
temperature, followed by bleeding from her nose and the
venepuncture sites. A coagulation profile shows an elevated
APTT, PT and thrombin time; her D-dimer level is raised; and
there is an associated thrombocytopenia.

Theme: **Haemolytic anaemia**

Options

A   G6PD deficiency
B   Hereditary spherocytosis
C   Microangiopathic haemolytic
    anaemia
D   Paroxysmal cold
    haemoglobinuria

E   Paroxysmal nocturnal
    haemoglobinuria
F   Pyruvate kinase deficiency
G   Sickle cell anaemia
H   Thalassaemia
I   Warm autoimmune haemolytic
    anaemia

Instructions

For each of the patients described below choose the SINGLE most likely diagnosis from the list of options above. Each option may be used once, more than once or not at all.

150 A 55-year-old man initially presented to his doctor complaining of feeling generally unwell and lethargic. He also admitted to intermittent episodes of dark-coloured urine. Tests show he is anaemic and his GP has prescribed iron therapy. □

151 A 26-year-old man had a full blood count done as a part of routine screening and was found to have a haemoglobin of 5 g/dl and a raised reticulocyte count. There was a positive family history. The oxygen dissociation curve was shifted to the right, which explained the lack of symptoms. A peripheral blood film showed prickle cells. Over the next few years he required multiple transfusions, especially during episodes of infection. His condition has improved following splenectomy. □

152 A 16-year-old of African descent has been referred to you after presenting to his GP with recurrent episodes of severe pain in his legs, especially in the dorsum of his feet. During some of these episodes he developed haematuria with evidence of haemolysis, which was greater during episodes of concurrent infection. He is especially prone to *Streptococcus pneumoniae* infection. His blood film shows features of hyposplenism. □

153 A 24-year-old man presented to his GP with a dragging pain in his left hypochondrium. Examination revealed splenomegaly. FBC shows haemolytic anaemia. He also has ulcers on his left shin. Gallbladder stones are evident on USS of his abdomen. A direct Coombs' test is negative.   ☐

Theme: **Treatment of epilepsy**

Options

A	Carbamazepine	G	Phenobarbital
B	Clobazam	H	Phenytoin
C	Clonazepam	I	Sodium valproate
D	Ethosuximide *2nd line for absence*	J	Tiagabine
E	Gabapentin	K	Topiramate
F	Lamotrigine *partial seizures*		

Instructions

For each of the patients described below choose the SINGLE most useful drug from the list of options above. Each option may be used once, more than once or not at all.

154 A 46-year-old man was diagnosed with partial seizures. He is obese, with a BMI of 44. He was initially put on carbamazepine; he is now on sodium valproate, but with poor control of seizures. ☐

155 A 26-year-old woman taking the OCP developed what has been diagnosed as absence or petit mal seizures. ☐

156 A 10-year-old child with petit mal seizures was started on sodium valproate but this had to be stopped due to liver dysfunction. The child has since continued to have absence seizures. A second medication is prescribed. ☐

157 A patient developed epileptic cluster attacks, which were more frequent during menstruation. The attacks decreased in number when she was started on valproic acid but still continued. As an adjunct to valproic acid, she is now taking a drug that can be used as a short-term 'off and on' agent. ☐

Medicine EMQs – Answers

Theme: **Investigation of respiratory disease**

1 **H: Transfer factor**
The transfer factor will be increased in this case, which, though not diagnostic, is a classic manifestation and does point to the diagnosis. CXR, HRCT and bleeding on bronchoscopy will clinch the diagnosis.

2 **D: Mediastinoscopy**
A transbronchial biopsy is usually the best investigation for obtaining a tissue diagnosis. Next to that, mediastinoscopy, although more invasive, would also help towards a tissue diagnosis.

3 **A: CT PA**
A computed tomography pulmonary angiogram has been recommended by the British Thoracic Society as the investigation of choice in any patient with a suspected pulmonary embolism (PE). However, in this scenario a ventilation–perfusion scan would also be quite effective.

4 **E: Pleural biopsy**
A pleural biopsy will give a definite diagnosis. Unfortunately, the yield is not very high with a blind biopsy and a medical thoracoscopic biopsy or a biopsy at open surgery is often necessary to clinch the diagnosis.

5 **G: Skin-prick test**
Allergic bronchopulmonary aspergillosis (ABPA) is diagnosed by, among other things, skin-prick testing to protein allergens from *Aspergillus fumigatus*. This results in immediately positive skin tests.

Theme: Management of obstructive airways
diseases

6   C: Fluticasone
The British Thoracic Society (BTS) guidelines and the National
Institute for Clinical Excellence (NICE) guidelines recommend
the use of steroid inhalers in patients with severe COPD and
repeated hospitalisations, irrespective of lung function
parameters.

7   K: Tiotropium
Tiotropium, a long-acting anticholinergic agent, has been found
to bring about a marked improvement in quality of life and
reduce the number of hospital admissions for patients with
moderate to severe COPD. It cannot, however, be used in
conjunction with ipratropium.

8   E: Long-term oxygen therapy
Oxygen is the only agent that has been shown to improve survival
in patients with severe COPD and cor pulmonale.

9   L: Zafirlukast
This leukotriene antagonist has been shown to improve the
control of asthma when used in step 4 of the 'stepladder'
treatment of asthma.

10   J: Salmeterol
Salmeterol has been shown to be very effective in controlling the
nocturnal awakenings in people with asthma. It acts better when
used in conjunction with a steroid inhaler.

11   F: Magnesium sulphate
This has been recommended as the agent of choice for treating
patients with acute severe asthma who have failed to respond to
nebulisation.

Theme: Pneumonia

12   C: *Legionella pneumophila*
A strong presumptive diagnosis of *Legionella* is possible in the majority of patients when three of the following four features are present: a prodromal viral illness; a dry cough, confusion or diarrhoea; lymphopenia without marked leucocytosis; hyponatraemia.

13   B: *Klebsiella pneumoniae*
Pneumonia occurs in elderly patients who have pre-existing co-morbidity. Upper lobe cavitating lesions are common, with bulging of the fissures. This organism can be found in sputum and in blood cultures.

14   F: *Pseudomonas aeruginosa*
The presence of this organism correlates with a worsening clinical condition and higher mortality in patients with cystic fibrosis.

15   D: *Mycoplasma pneumoniae*
Infection with this organism may result in cough and dramatic X-ray appearances, which may last for weeks. Patients can relapse. Extrapulmonary complications can occur at any time in the course of the illness.

16   E: *Pneumocystis jiroveci*
In contrast to infection with *Mycoplasma*, the clinical features of PJP (formerly known as *Pneumocystis carinii* (PCP)) are far worse than the radiological appearances. In 90% of cases the diagnosis can be made by using indirect immunofluorescence with monoclonal antibodies to stain the sputum.

Theme: Diseases of the respiratory system

17   G: Progressive massive fibrosis
PMF occurs in 30% of patients with a background of category 3 simple pneumoconiosis. They have considerable effort-dyspnoea, which may progress even after exposure to coal dust has ceased.

18   F: Motor neurone disease
Any cause of bilateral diaphragmatic weakness or paralysis causes

a decrease in tidal volume and an increased respiratory rate. Sniffing causes a paradoxical inward movement of the abdominal wall, best seen in the supine position.

19   B: Churg–Strauss syndrome

This syndrome occurs in males, with a triad of rhinitis and asthma, eosinophilia and systemic vasculitis. It typically involves the lungs, peripheral nerves and skin, but spares the kidneys. The disease responds well to corticosteroid treatment.

20   D: Extrinsic allergic alveolitis

Continued exposure will lead to features of fibrosing alveolitis. Prevention is the aim. Prednisolone in high doses will lead to the regression of the disease in the early stages.

Theme: Lung cancer

21   H: Squamous-cell carcinoma

This is now categorised within 'non-small-cell lung cancer'. Squamous-cell carcinoma is the type of lung cancer most closely associated with smoking. Along with causing hypertrophic pulmonary osteoarthropathy (HPOA), it is also the commonest type of cancer that gives rise to hypercalcaemia. Squamous-cell carcinomas are responsive to radiotherapy but are relatively chemoresistant. Surgery is beneficial in patients with a peripheral non-small-cell lung cancer.

22   B: Alveolar-cell carcinoma

This type of carcinoma comprises 1–2% of lung tumours. Alveolar-cell carcinomas can be diffuse, nodular, multicentric lesions.

23   A: Adenocarcinoma

An adenocarcinoma most commonly occurs as a subpleural mass. Adenocarcinomas account for 10% of all lung cancers. They are proportionally more common in non-smokers, the very elderly and in Far Eastern populations. It is also classified as a 'non-small-cell cancer'.

24   G: Small-cell carcinoma

Small-cell carcinomas are responsible for most paraneoplastic syndromes, because of the secretion of many polypeptide hormones from endocrine cells (Kultchitsky cells). They are chemosensitive but have a high recurrence rate. This is considered to be more of a systemic disease.

25   F: Pulmonary hamartoma
This is the most common benign tumour of the lung. Although this tumour is usually extremely slow-growing, it may reach a large size. It is usually found as an incidental finding on chest X-ray.

26   C: Bronchial carcinoid
A bronchial carcinoid is locally invasive. Eventually, it may involve mediastinal lymph nodes and then metastasise to distant organs. It grows slowly, eventually blocking the bronchus and leading to lobar collapse.

NB. This question may appear in a clinical scenario. However, remembering these facts will be very relevant to answering questions about lung cancer.

Theme: Gastrointestinal bleeding

27   M: Ulcerative colitis
This disease can be mild, moderate or severe. Although it can follow a chronic course in 10% of patients, some will only have one attack. The symptoms in the scenario will generally occur with proctitis and few systemic manifestations.

28   H: Ischaemic colitis
On examination the abdomen is often distended and tender. A straight abdominal X-ray shows thumb-printing at the site of the splenic flexure. The differential diagnosis is acute colitis.

29   D: Dieulafoy's gastric vascular abnormality
Endoscopic diagnosis of extragastric Dieulafoy's lesion can be difficult because of its small size and obscure location. Increased awareness and careful and early endoscopic evaluation following the bleeding episode are the key to accurate diagnosis. Endoscopic adrenaline (epinephrine) injection is one of the important treatment modalities for the control of bleeding.

30 L: Pseudoxanthoma elasticum
PXE is rare, only occurring in about 1 in 160,000 of the general
population. Arterial inelasticity can lead to bleeding from the
gastrointestinal tract and, rarely, acute vomiting of blood.

31 I: Mallory–Weiss syndrome
Mallory–Weiss syndrome is haematemesis from a tear in the
mucosa of the oesophagus, brought on by prolonged vomiting
due to a variety of causes. The tear most often develops in the
lower oesophagus, close to the oesophagogastric junction.
Melaena may develop later. It may occur as a result of
alcohol-related vomiting or the recurrent morning sickness of
pregnancy. This syndrome must not be confused with Boerhaave's
syndrome (where there is a spontaneous perforation of a
non-diseased oesophagus) or with an intramural rupture.

Theme: Malabsorption

32 B: Coeliac disease
Other manifestations may include tetany, osteomalacia, and even
gross malnutrition leading to peripheral oedema. Polyneuropathy
and paraesthesia may also occur.

33 A: Bacterial overgrowth
The normal terminal ileum contains faecal-type organisms such
as *Escherichia coli* and various anaerobes. Bacterial overgrowth
usually only occurs in association with a structural abnormality of
the small intestine. However, it may occasionally present in the
very elderly in the absence of such abnormality.

34 H: Whipple's disease
The heart, lung and brain may also be involved in patients with
Whipple's disease. Histologically, the villi are stunted and contain
diagnostic PAS-positive macrophages.

35 D: *Giardia* infestation
The causative organism can be found in jejunal fluid or mucosa.

Theme: Diseases of the small intestine

36 E: Intestinal lymphangiectasia
Lymphatic dilatation may be primary or secondary to lymphatic obstruction, as in constrictive pericarditis or malignancy.

37 A: Abetalipoproteinaemia
This is due to a failure of apo B-100 synthesis in the liver and apo B-48 in the intestinal cells, with the result that chylomicrons are not formed.

38 J: Tuberculosis
The diagnosis here is of intestinal TB, the increasing incidence of which is related to HIV infection.

39 C: Eosinophilic gastroenteritis
Eosinophilia is present in 20% of such cases. Radiology or endoscopy will demonstrate the lesion.

40 H: Small intestinal ischaemia
The diagnosis is made by angiogram.

Theme: Colonic disorders

41 A: Crohn's disease
Barium enemas have been superseded by CT colonoscopy for diagnosing colonic disease. Spiral CT scans are useful for delineating abscesses, masses and thickened bowel. Ultrasound is useful for demonstrating masses and also in follow-up.

42 H: Ulcerative colitis
An early change in UC is aphthoid ulceration, while deep ulceration occurs in late stages. Disease activity can be assessed from the clinical picture and laboratory tests: erythrocyte sedimentation rate (ESR), serum albumin and acute-phase reactants (C-reactive protein (CRP) or orosomucoids). In some centres, areas of localised inflammation are assessed by the presence of radiolabelled leucocytes injected intravenously.

43 F: Megacolon

A preliminary rectal biopsy is stained for the presence of ganglion cells in the submucous plexus.

44 B: Diverticulitis

An ultrasound scan (USS) can demonstrate a thickened bowel and large pericolic collection. It is less sensitive than CT.

45 G: Pneumatosis cystoides intestinalis

The investigations are aimed at demonstrating the cysts. Continuous oxygen therapy will help to disperse the large oxygen-containing cysts.

NB. This question may appear in a clinical scenario. However, remembering these facts will be very relevant to answering questions about colonic cancer. Questions just on radiology and histology, while uncommon, are definitely not unheard of!

Theme: Diarrhoea

46 I: Purgative abuse

Commonly seen in women, patients are usually extensively investigated for chronic diarrhoea. Melanosis coli may also be seen in people regularly taking laxatives at normal doses for long periods. In advanced cases, a barium enema may show loss of the haustral pattern and a dilated colon.

47 A: Behçet's disease

Except for ocular attacks, all the common manifestations of this disease are self-limiting. Repeated attacks of uveitis can lead to blindness. The pathergy reaction is highly specific to Behçet's disease.

48 B: *Campylobacter* diarrhoea

Invasive haemorrhagic colitis is sometimes seen. Diagnosis is made on the results of stool cultures. Ciprofloxacin may be required for the treatment of severe cases.

49   E: Irritable bowel syndrome
The pain is classically situated in the left iliac fossa and is relieved by defecation and the passage of wind. Stools are ribbon-like and 'rabbity' in appearance. Diarrhoea indicates organic disease. Air insufflation on sigmoidoscopy can sometimes reproduce the pain.

50   F: Medullary carcinoma of the thyroid
All compressive symptoms associated with thyroid cancer may be found. Local invasion and metastasis is common. Although the tumour responds slowly to treatment, progression is slow.

Theme: **Diagnosis of connective tissue disorders**

51   E: Polymyositis
ANA (antinuclear antibody) is commonly positive in patients with polymyositis, while rheumatoid factor is positive in only 50% of cases. Anti-Jo-1 antibodies are predictive of pulmonary fibrosis but are rarely present in dermatomyositis. MRI is used to target abnormal muscle. Screening for malignancy is limited to relatively non-invasive techniques.

52   B: Limited cutaneous scleroderma
Speckled, nucleolar and anticentromere antibodies occur in 70–80% of cases.

53   H: Systemic lupus erythematosus
Serum ANAs are positive in almost all cases. Double-stranded DNA (dsDNA) binding is specific for SLE, although it is found in only 50% of cases. Rheumatoid factor is present in 25% of cases. Immunoglobulin levels are raised.

54   G: Sjögren's syndrome
ANA are present in 60–70% cases and AMA (antimitochondrial antibody) in 10%. Anti-Ro antibodies are present in 70% of patients and are of particular interest because they can cross the placenta and can cause complete heart block in the fetus.

Theme: **Presentation of autoimmune diseases**

55 H: Systemic lupus erythematosus
This is an inflammatory multisystem disorder with arthralgia and
rashes being the most common manifestations; cerebral and renal
disease are the most serious problems. The heart is involved in
25% of cases. Pericarditis and small pericardial effusions detected
by echocardiography are common. Aortic valve lesions and
cardiomyopathy can occur, albeit rarely. A non-infective
endocarditis involving the mitral valve (Libman–Sacks syndrome)
is very rare.

56 G: Sjögren's syndrome
The presence of dry eyes in the absence of rheumatoid arthritis
(RA) or any other autoimmune disease is called 'primary
Sjögren's syndrome'. Other associated manifestations include
dysphagia and abnormal oesophageal motility, pulmonary
fibrosis, polyneuropathy, vasculitis and an increased incidence of
non-Hodgkin's lymphoma.

57 A: Antiphospholipid antibody syndrome
The antiphospholipid antibody syndrome is associated with
negatively charged antibodies to phospholipids. Patients with this
syndrome are also known to have abortions, chorea, migraine,
livedo reticularis and a positive Coombs' test.

58 I: Systemic sclerosis
The skin is initially oedematous and then becomes tight. Several
months later the patient develops Raynaud's phenomenon.
Oesophageal problems cause heartburn and reflux, and there may
be malabsorption due to bacterial overgrowth and dilatation of
the small bowel. Renal involvement is due to obliterative
endarteritis causing renal failure and malignant hypertension.
Lung fibrosis is the most common cause of death.

Theme: **Inflammatory arthritis**

59 A: Ankylosing spondylitis
The disease occurs more often in men than women (25:1), and is

milder in women than in men. In young teenage boys, lower limb monoarthritis may pre-date the development of spinal problems. Acute anterior uveitis is strongly related to HLA-B27.

60   F: Psoriatic arthropathy

Although psoriatic arthritis is less severe than rheumatoid arthritis, it is unsightly, resulting in sausage-like fingers and toes. Arthritis mutilans affects 5% of people. Only 50% are positive for HLA-B27.

61   G: Reactive arthritis

Some 70% patients recover fully within 6 months but many relapse. The classic triad of Reiter's disease is urethritis, arthritis and conjunctivitis.

62   C: Gout

Gout is characterised by hyperuricaemia due to the overproduction (75%) or under-excretion (25%) of uric acid. Causes of impaired excretion include chronic renal failure, drug therapy (thiazide diuretics, low-dose aspirin), hypertension and lead toxicity. Increased production of uric acid is caused by Lesch–Nyhan syndrome (hypoxanthine-guanine phosphoribosyltransferase (HGPRT) deficiency) and phosphoribosyl pyrophosphate transferase (PRPPT) overactivity, polycythaemia vera and leukaemia, among others. Since both HGPRT and PRPPT are involved in purine metabolic pathways, patients with gout should avoid purine-rich foods, such as offal, sardines and shellfish, legumes and alcohol. Untreated attacks can last for up to 7 days.

63   D: Lyme's arthritis

Patients develop a fever and a headache with an expanding erythematous rash called 'erythema chronicum migrans'. About 25% of patients develop an acute pauciarticular arthritis.

Theme: **Imaging techniques for renal diseases**

64   I: Renal scintigraphy

After the injection of, for example [$^{99}Tc^m$]MAG3 (mercaptoacetyl triglycine), a rise in resistance to pelvic or ureteric flow prolongs the parenchymal transit time of the tracer, usually leading to a delay in emptying the pelvis. Whereas an obstructive uropathy is associated with a prolonged transit of tracer through the renal parenchyma, a normal parenchymal transit time with delayed outflow indicates a non-obstructed dilated pelvis.

65 D: Micturating cystography
The patient is screened during voiding after a contrast agent has been instilled into the bladder. This is to check for vesicoureteric reflux and to study urethral and bladder emptying.

66 B: CT scan
First-line uses of CT scan include: characterisation of renal masses that are indeterminate on USS (ultrasound screening); staging of renal tumours; detection of lucent calculi; evaluation of the retroperitoneum for tumours or fibrosis; assessment of renal trauma; and visualisation of renal arteries and veins.

67 K: USS
This investigation is also useful for checking whether renal masses are solid or cystic, detecting intrarenal or perinephric fluid, and for demonstrating renal perfusion.

NB. This is another situation where a clinical scenario can be used in conjunction with the investigational modality. However, the questions may well be posed as here. They are useful learning points and should be remembered.

Theme: **Diagnosis of renal diseases**

68 A: Acute tubulointerstitial nephritis
Many of these patients have eosinophilia and eosinophiluria. Renal biopsy shows intense interstitial cellular infiltrate. High-dose steroid therapy is often given, but its efficacy has not been proved.

69 H: Thrombotic thrombocytopenic purpura
HUS is characterised by intravascular haemolysis and red cell fragmentation, thrombocytopenia and acute renal failure. TTP, on the other hand, characteristically involves microangiopathic haemolysis, renal failure and neurological disturbances.

70 F: Medullary cystic kidney disease
Progressive glomerular failure is a secondary event. The cysts are rarely visualised by imaging techniques.

71 G: Retroperitoneal fibrosis
The condition may extend from the level of the second lumbar vertebra to the pelvic brim. The close differential diagnosis is retroperitoneal lymphoma.

Theme: Management of renal failure

72 K: Oral phosphodiesterase inhibitors
Sildenafil has been shown to be effective in controlled trials of patients with end-stage renal failure. Coronary artery disease and treatment with nitrates are known contraindications to this treatment.

73 G: Haemofiltration
This patient needs 'invasive' treatment in spite of his co-morbidity. Because his stoma will make the successful placement of a catheter very unlikely, haemodialysis rather than peritoneal dialysis is the modality of choice.

74 E: Catheterisation
This patient's symptoms and biochemistry are consistent with acute urinary retention, which might have been precipitated by the administration of a diuretic for his suspected heart failure. Catheterisation must, however, be accompanied by adequate hydration to keep his electrolyte balance intact.

75 I: Intravenous fluid
A large volume of fluid loss without adequate replacement can often result in prerenal failure, which, however, can be corrected by judicious fluid replacement.

76 C: Calcium resonium
In some instances, just stopping the medications may lower potassium levels. However, if this is unsuccessful, an ion-exchange resin may work; but dialysis may be needed. In patients with a prolonged rise of their serum potassium level, acute measures are neither useful nor necessary.

Theme: **Treatment of cardiac arrhythmias**

77 A: Amiodarone

Amiodarone is used to suppress and treat cardiac arrhythmias, both ventricular and supraventricular. Given intravenously it is effective in suppressing serious arrhythmias. Given over a long period of time by mouth, it effectively suppresses life-threatening ventricular arrhythmias, and also chronic atrial fibrillation. Amiodarone is of particular value in patients who have severe arrhythmias due to accessory pathways (Wolff–Parkinson–White syndrome). Strong contraindications include: second- or third-degree AV block (unless paced), severe bradycardia, pregnancy, breast-feeding (excreted in breast milk).

78 B: Cardiac pacemaker

Complete heart block or second degree heart block which is symptomatic in the form of syncope, and sick sinus syndrome are some of the indications for permanent pacemaker insertion.

79 E: Flecainide

In the stable patient with acute-onset atrial fibrillation and uncompromised left ventricular function, flecainide is the most efficacious drug at restoring normal sinus rhythm expediently. However, approximately 60% of patients will revert with no treatment.

80 G: Metoprolol

Initially up to 5 mg injected iv at a rate of 1–2 mg per minute. The injection can be repeated at 5-minute intervals until a satisfactory response has been obtained. A total dose of 10–15 mg generally proves sufficient. Because of the risk of a pronounced drop of blood pressure, the iv administration of metoprolol to patients with a systolic blood pressure below 100 mmHg should only be given with special care.

NB. In general, Class Ic agents are used to treat patients with no significant heart disease, and Class III agents are preferred in patients with significant structural heart disease. Younger patients with lone paroxysmal AF should be assessed to rule out a single atrial ectopic focus triggering AF: this form of AF can be effectively cured by catheter ablation. For non-sustained VT, β-blocker therapy is an initial safe choice for symptom relief in most patients.

Theme: Results of cardiac investigations

81   C: Constrictive pericarditis
CXR shows a relatively small heart; a lateral film reveals obvious calcification.

82   B: Atrial septal defect
Subcostal views usually demonstrate the defect. The CXR will show prominent pulmonary artery and pulmonary plethora.

83   F: Mitral valve prolapse
Contrast angiogram performed during cardiac catheterisation reveals systolic prolapse of the mitral valve into the left atrium, and, if present, mitral regurgitation will be seen. This investigation is not normally required, however.

84   D: HOCM
Certain mutations, for example of the troponin gene, can be associated with no hypertrophy. Family history analysis reveals an autosomal dominant mode of inheritance.

85   A: Atrial myxoma
Myxomas can occur in the ventricles or in the right atrium. The tumour can obstruct the mitral valve, or may be the site of thrombi, which can then embolise.

Theme: Viral illness

86   I: Yellow fever virus
The mortality rate from infection with this virus is about 40%. The diagnosis is established by taking a careful history of the patient's travel and vaccination status, and by isolating the virus from a blood sample during the first 3 days of illness. Treatment is supportive.

87   H: Rubella virus
The petechial lesions on the soft palate are called 'Forchheimer spots'. Complications are rare, but include superadded pulmonary bacterial infections, arthralgia, haemorrhagic manifestations due to thrombocytopenia, encephalitis and the congenital rubella syndrome.

88 G: Poliovirus

Paralytic polio occurs in about 13% of infected adults. The features initially resemble those of abortive polio, but, in adults, they usually progress to quadriparesis. President Roosevelt, himself a polio sufferer, declared war on polio. During the 1950s, an intensified research effort, using monkeys, rats and mice, resulted in the development of the Sabin and Salk polio vaccines. Because of these, polio is now virtually unknown in the USA and Europe and the vaccines are estimated to have already prevented over two million cases of polio.

89 E: Epstein–Barr virus

EBV is strongly suspected if atypical mononuclear cells are found on a peripheral blood smear. According to Harrison's and to Kumar and Clark's textbooks of medicine, the Paul–Bunnell reaction becomes positive during the second week of infection. This test detects heterophile antibodies (IgM) that agglutinate sheep erythrocytes. However, false-positives can occur in patients with viral hepatitis, Hodgkin's disease or acute leukaemia.

NB. Candidates should familiarise themselves with the latest GMC recommendations for standard immunisations in children and adults.

Theme: **Bacterial illness**

90 G: Plague

The diagnosis is established by demonstrating the organism (*Yersinia pestis*) in a lymph node aspirate. Although chloramphenicol can be used, the first-line treatment is now oral tetracycline or im streptomycin. Plague is endemic in many countries: in Africa, the Americas and Asia. In 1999, 14 countries reported 2603 cases to the WHO (including 212 deaths). These figures are comparable with the annual average figures (2547 cases, 181 deaths) for the previous 10 years (1988–1997). Over the past decade, 76.2% of all cases and 81.8% of all deaths were reported from Africa.

91 **B: Anthrax**

This is the cutaneous variety, as opposed to the more severe respiratory variant (the latter is also known as 'woolsorters' disease' since the causative agent, a strain of *Bacillus anthracis*, could be inhaled from the fleece of infected sheep). Transmission is by direct contact with an infected animal. Diagnosis is reached by demonstrating the organism on a smear or in culture, or by serological testing.

92 **C: Leprosy**

This description is absolutely classic of lepromatous leprosy (LL). The face, gluteal region and extremities are most commonly associated. Nerve involvement leads to muscle atrophy. Patients with tuberculoid leprosy (TL) have a single hypopigmented skin lesion. Treatment for borderline (BB), borderline lepromatous (BL) or LL – the multibacillary form – is triple therapy with dapsone + clofazimine + rifampicin. Patients with tuberculoid (TT) and borderline tuberculoid (BT) forms of leprosy are treated monthly with dapsone + rifampicin for a total of 6 months.

93 **D: Leptospirosis**

The diagnosis is usually a clinical one. The organism (*Leptospira interrogans*, of which there are various serotypes) can be cultured from blood or CSF in the first week of illness. The organism can also be detected by polymerase chain reaction and by an enzyme-linked immunosorbent assay (ELISA). Specific IgM antibodies start to appear from the end of the first week of illness. Treatment is with oral doxycycline in mild cases and iv penicillin in severe cases.

Theme: **Fungal and protozoal illnesses**

94 **D: Coccidioidomycosis**

Because of the high infectivity of the fungus, and consequent risk to laboratory personnel, serological tests are widely used for diagnosis. Ketoconazole or itraconazole for 6 months is the treatment of choice for primary pulmonary disease.

95   I: Malaria

Falciparum malaria is the most severe form of malaria, with high levels of parasitaemia. The infected red blood cells develop peculiar knob-like fenestrations that facilitate their adhesion to the endothelium of the blood vessel. The consequent vascular occlusion causes anoxic organ damage, mainly of the kidney, liver, brain and gastrointestinal tract. Quinine, given by slow intravenous infusion, is the drug of choice.

96   C: Chagas' disease

Acute infection occurring in children usually passes unnoticed. A firm, reddish papule occurs at the site of entry of infection. In the case of conjunctival infection, the eyes will be swollen and the eyelids will close – Romaña's sign. After a latent period of many years some people may develop a chronic infection. Death occurs in a small proportion of patients due to myocarditis and meningoencephalitis. More commonly, patients recover completely in a few weeks. Nifurtimox was widely used to treat acute disease but is no longer produced. Benzimidazole for 60 days is now the treatment of choice.

97   F: Giardiasis

Giardia lamblia causes small intestinal disease with diarrhoea and malabsorption. There is evidence that morphological damage to the small intestine may be immune-mediated. Metronidazole or tinidazole are the drugs of choice.

Theme: **Chronic immunodeficiency syndromes**

98   C: Chronic granulomatous disease   _X– linked recessive_

Infections respond to appropriate antimicrobial therapy and surgical treatment. Regular interferon-γ can reduce the frequency of infections.

99   B: Chédiak–Higashi syndrome   _Autosomal recessive_

A defect of branchial arch development leads to abnormal thymic development. The absent thymus can be documented radiologically.

Di George!

100   H: Wiskott–Aldrich syndrome
This is mainly a cell-mediated defect, with falling immunoglobulin levels and autoimmune defects.

101   G: Severe combined immunodeficiency
Bone marrow transplantation is the definitive treatment, and is significantly successful.

Theme: **Vitamin deficiency**

102   F: Vitamin C
The type of anaemia associated with vitamin C deficiency is generally hypochromic. A low plasma ascorbic acid level clinches the diagnosis.

103   A: Niacin
Symptoms of minor niacin deficiency are tiredness, depression and loss of memory. The disease pellagra results from a severe deficiency of niacin, and is characterised by the three D's – **diarrhoea, dermatitis and dementia**. Niacin deficiency is common in certain maize-eating populations because the niacin in maize (and other cereal grains) is bound in such a way as to make it unavailable to the body. To compound this problem, maize is also a relatively poor source of tryptophan.

104   D: Vitamin B_1
The diagnosis is confirmed by measuring transketolase activity in red cells using fresh heparinised blood.

105   B: Riboflavin
Riboflavin deficiency usually occurs in conjunction with deficiencies of the other water-soluble vitamins. Specific symptoms of riboflavin deficiency include: glossitis (magenta tongue), angular stomatitis (fissures at the corner of the mouth), itching and a skin rash.

NB. All manifestations of single vitamin deficiencies can actually be mimicked by combined vitamin deficiences, but such an option does not appear in the list. In answering EMQs and SBAs you go for the nearest correct answer.

Theme: **Skin disorders**

106   D: Lichen planus

Although this condition often clears after 18 months, it may recur. Ulcerative mucosal disease is often premalignant. The condition requires the use of potent topical steroids and oral prednisolone.

107   E: Pityriasis rosea

The long axis of the oval lesions tends to run along dermatomal lines, giving rise to a 'Christmas tree' appearance on the patient's back. This is preceded by the appearance of a 'herald patch'.

108   C: Guttate psoriasis

Guttate psoriasis is a distinctive acute form of psoriasis that characteristically occurs in children and young adults. It is closely associated with a preceding streptococcal sore throat or tonsillitis. Some authorities have claimed that ordinary (chronic plaque) psoriasis may also be made worse by infection at distant sites. Although many dermatologists have recommended using antibiotics to treat guttate psoriasis in particular, it is unclear whether they influence the course of either form of psoriasis. Some dermatologists have also recommended tonsillectomy to treat psoriasis in patients with recurrent streptococcal sore throats.

109   B: Granuloma annulare

The pathology shows a granulomatous dermal infiltrate with foci of collagen degeneration. Spontaneous resolution occurs, but triamcinolone injection or cryotherapy helps localised disease.

Theme: **Treatment for parkinsonism**

110   C: Benzatropine

The acute dystonic reactions that sometimes occur with neuroleptics respond promptly to iv benzatropine.

111   F: Levodopa + benserazide
Approaches to treatment include: shortening the interval between levodopa doses, adding in selegiline, adding in dopaminergic agonists, and using entacapone or drug holidays.

112   I: Stereotactic surgery
When successful, surgery provides effective, if temporary, improvement in tremor and dyskinesia. Thalamic stimulation is also used.

113   B: Apomorphine
A subcutaneous apomorphine pump is an effective way to smooth out the responses to fluctuations in levodopa levels. However, vomiting is a problem and haemolytic anaemia is a rare side-effect.

Theme: Investigations for CNS disorders

114   E: Guillain–Barré syndrome
The diagnosis of GBS is established on clinical grounds and confirmed by nerve conduction studies. CSF protein is typically elevated, but both the cell count and sugar level are normal.

115   G: Multiple sclerosis
With diagnostic magnetic resonance images and a compatible clinical picture, a CSF examination is often unnecessary.

116   I: Narcolepsy
Narcolepsy attacks are periods of irresistible sleep, ie excessive daytime drowsiness, in inappropriate circumstances. Episodes tend to occur when there is little distraction.

117   H: Myasthenia gravis
The Tensilon® test may also be used to diagnose this condition. A CXR may show a thymoma. Although a muscle biopsy is not usually performed, it would show ultrastructural abnormalities.

Theme: CNS disorders

118 G: Syringomyelia
This is usually associated with Arnold–Chiari malformations.
Due to an anatomical abnormality at the foramen magnum,
normal pulsatile CSF pressure waves are transmitted to the
fragile structures within the cervical cord and brainstem, thus
causing secondary cavity formation. There are areas of
dissociated sensory loss, neuropathic joints and brainstem signs.

119 D: Idiopathic intracranial hypertension
This condition was once called 'pseudotumour cerebri'. There is
neither a mass nor an increase in ventricular size. Imaging is
normal. Thiazide diuretics and acetazolamide reduce the
intracranial pressure seen in this condition.

120 B: Creutzfeldt–Jakob disease
Patients with variant CJD (vCJD) are younger than patients with
the sporadic disease, with a mean age of 29 years. Early
symptoms are neuropsychiatric.

121 H: Tabes dorsalis
The cause is demyelination of the posterior roots.

122 C: Huntington's disease
Relentlessly progressive dementia and chorea, usually occurring
in middle life, but sometimes in childhood, are the hallmarks of
this inherited fatal disease. There is a progressive loss of small
neurones in the putamen and caudate nucleus.

123 A: Cortical venous thrombosis
Cerebral venous thrombosis is a rare disorder with highly
variable and non-specific clinical presentations. The mainstay of
treatment is anticoagulation with heparin, even in the case of
cerebral haemorrhage, followed as soon as possible by oral
anticoagulant administration.

Theme: Typical stroke syndromes

124 C: Lateral medullary syndrome
This is also called 'posterior inferior cerebellar artery
thrombosis' and 'Wallenberg's syndrome'.

125   B: Binswanger's disease
This is an imaging term describing low-attenuation areas in the cerebral white matter on CT, with dementia, TIA and stroke episodes in hypertensive patients.

126   I: Weber's syndrome
This is due to a lesion in one half of the midbrain.

127   D: Locked-in syndrome
'Locked in' syndrome is the result of a bilateral lesion in the medulla due to occlusion of the penetrating midline branches of the basilar artery. Characteristically, the patient is unable to talk, swallow or move the limbs despite being conscious and alert. Some facial and eye movements are preserved, permitting elementary communication. Spinothalamic sensation is retained but discriminatory sensation in the limbs is lost due to damage to the medial lemniscus. The prognosis is poor.

Theme: Endocrine diseases

128   E: Hashimoto's thyroiditis
Thyroid function tests show an initial hyperthyroidism. Thyroid uptake scans show suppression of uptake during the acute phase. Hypothyroidism, though usually transient, may follow after a few weeks.

129   D: Ectopic ACTH-producing tumour
This is distinguished by a short history, pigmentation and weight loss, unprovoked hypokalaemia and diabetes and plasma ACTH levels of 200 ng/l. However, many ectopic tumours are benign and closely mimic pituitary disease, both clinically and biochemically.

130   A: Conn's syndrome
The classic features are hypokalaemia, urinary potassium loss of more than 30 mmol/day during hypokalaemia, an elevated plasma aldosterone:renin ratio and an elevated plasma aldosterone that is not suppressed by a 0.9% saline or fludrocortisone infusion.

131   H: Phaeochromocytoma
Measurement of urinary metanephrines (metabolites of

epinephrine (ie adrenaline)) and plasma and urinary
catecholamines, and clonidine suppression and glucagon
stimulation tests may be appropriate.

Theme: Overdoses

132   D: Carbon monoxide
Methylene chloride, which is present in many paint strippers, is
metabolised to carbon monoxide. The treatment would be to
remove the patient from the source and then to administer
high-flow oxygen through a tightly fitting face mask.
Endotracheal intubation and mechanical ventilation would be
required for the unconscious patient.

133   G: Theophylline
There is good evidence that multiple-dose activated charcoal
enhances theophylline excretion. A non-selective β-blocker (eg
propranolol) is useful in the treatment of tachyarrhythmias
secondary to hypokalaemia. Vomiting in an adult should be
suppressed by iv ondansetron.

134   F: Organophosphate insecticides
Mild cases require no treatment other than the removal of soiled
clothing and washing of contaminated skin with soap and water.
Intravenous atropine and pralidoxime should be given to
symptomatic patients.

135   B: Aspirin
Charcoal lavage should be given if the ingestion has taken place
within an hour. The patient should receive an intravenous
transfusion (IVT) to correct dehydration and electrolyte
imbalance. Urinary alkalinisation should be carried out in
moderate overdose cases.

Theme: Common adverse effects of drugs in pregnancy

136   C: Methaemoglobinaemia and haemolysis in neonates
Chloroquine is embryotoxic and teratogenic in animals, causing
embryonic death, anophthalmia and micro-ophthalmia. In

humans, it crosses the human placenta. Although there have been no well-controlled human studies, there is a suggested possible association with an increased risk of malformations, including left-sided hemihypertrophy, cochleovestibular paresis and Wilms' tumour. Chloroquine is safe in breast-feeding, but is excreted into breast milk in amounts insufficient to protect the infant against malaria.

137   E: Neural tube defect

Carbamazepine crosses the placenta and is teratogenic in humans. It causes craniofacial and neural tube defects (mainly spina bifida), polydactyly, fingernail hypoplasia and developmental delay in infants exposed to the drug during the first trimester. There is also a suggested association with cardiovascular defects, absent gallbladder and thyroid gland, cleft lip, inguinal hernia, ambiguous genitalia, microcephaly and mental retardation in infants exposed during the first trimester. Although carbamazepine is excreted in small amounts into breast milk, it is safe for mothers to breast-feed.

138   B: Hare lip, cleft palate and cardiac abnormality

First trimester exposure to phenytoin causes the fetal hydantoin syndrome (FHS): craniofacial, limb and heart defects, oral clefts and impaired mental and physical growth. If given in association with phenobarbital, and amitriptyline, throughout pregnancy, it causes thanatophoric dwarfism. Anticonvulsant drugs, including phenytoin, can also cause haemorrhagic disease of the newborn by inducing thrombocytopenia or by suppressing vitamin K-dependent coagulation factors in the fetus. Phenytoin has been suggested to be a human transplacental carcinogen and infants exposed *in utero* may develop neuroblastoma, extrarenal Wilms' tumour, lymphangioma, ganglioneuroblastoma, ependymoblastoma, mesenchymoma or melanotic neuroectodermal tumours. Teratogenicity of the drug may be dose-related and so the lowest effective dose should be used for maintenance therapy during pregnancy.

However, it is known that phenytoin causes maternal folic acid deficiency, and therefore some of the neural tube deficits in the fetus could in fact be due to maternal folic acid deficiency rather than to the direct effect of phenytoin. Hence, women taking phenytoin who wish to become pregnant should be given adequate folic acid supplementation preconception and at least for the first trimester so that their folic acid level reaches that recommended for women who are not taking this antiepileptic drug.

Although phenytoin is excreted into breast milk, it is safe to breast-feed while taking therapeutic dosages. However, a single case of drowsiness, decreased suckling and methaemoglobinaemia has been reported in an infant exposed to phenytoin.

139   A: Damage to bones and teeth
Tetracycline crosses the placenta and, if used late in pregnancy, causes permanent tooth discoloration, enamel hypoplasia and impaired fetal skeletal growth. It also causes maternal fatty liver infiltration. Tetracycline is excreted into breast milk and, again, causes permanent tooth discoloration, enamel hypoplasia, impaired linear skeletal growth, oral and vaginal thrush and photosensitivity reactions.

Theme: **Haematological malignancies**

140   D: Chronic lymphoblastic leukaemia
The diagnosis is usually made on the peripheral blood film appearance, which shows typical small lymphocytes. Immunophenotyping confirms the diagnosis.

141   E: Hairy-cell leukaemia
Neoplastic disease of lymphoreticular cells is considered to be a rare type of chronic leukaemia. It is characterised by an insidious onset, splenomegaly, anaemia, granulocytopenia, thrombocytopenia, little or no lymphadenopathy, and the presence of hairy or flagellated cells in the blood and bone marrow.

142   F: Hodgkin's disease
The lymphomas represent an abnormal proliferation of B or T cells. A normocytic normochromic anaemia may be present. The erythrocyte sedimentation rate (ESR) is usually raised. Liver biochemistry is abnormal if the liver is involved. Chest X-ray

may show mediastinal involvement. A CT scan may show involvement of the intrathoracic, intra-abdominal and pelvic lymph nodes. In advanced disease, a bone marrow biopsy and trephine may show involvement. Lymph node biopsy will reveal the presence of Reed–Sternberg cells, which distinguishes this from non-Hodgkin's lymphoma.

143 C: Burkitt's lymphoma

Burkitt's lymphoma can be treated and cured, especially in children.

144 G: Myeloma

Myeloma is characterised by the presence of a serum paraprotein, which can be demonstrated as a monoclonal band on protein electrophoresis. The paraprotein is produced by abnormal proliferating plasma cells that generally produce IgG or IgA and, rarely, IgD. Anaemia and renal failure at presentation used to be two factors associated with a very poor prognosis: 50% of patients still die within 9 months.

145 J: Waldenström's macroglobulinaemia

There is pancytopenia, bone marrow aspiration shows infiltration with lymphoplasmacytoid cells and electrophoresis shows IgM paraprotein. Treatment is with alkylating agents.

Theme: **Coagulation disorders**

Blood changes in Haemophilia A, von Willebrand's disease and vitamin K deficiency

	Haemophilia A	von Willebrand's disease	Vitamin K deficiency
Bleeding time	Normal	↑	Normal
PT	Normal	Normal	↑
APTT	↑+	↑±	↑
Factor VIII:C	↓+	↓	Normal
vWF	Normal	↓	Normal

Key: ↑, increased; ↑+, much increased; ↑±, usually mildly increased; ↓, reduced; ↓+, much reduced. Abbreviations: PT, prothrombin time; APTT, activated partial thromboplastin time; vWF, von Willebrand factor.

146 D: Haemophilia A
See the table above.

147 H: von Willebrand's disease
See the table above.

148 G: Vitamin K deficiency
See the table above.

149 B: Disseminated intravascular coagulation
DIC is a condition in which the physiological generation of thrombin becomes unregulated. The unregulated generation of thrombin and plasmin results in the thrombotic and haemorrhagic features of DIC. The following list gives the laboratory features of DIC:

- thrombocytopenia: may be mild in chronic DIC
- elevated FDPs: fibrin degradation products may be measured by D-dimer assay (monoclonal antibodies to D-dimer fragments)
- fibrinogen: decreased in acute DIC; variable in chronic DIC
- PT: prothrombin time is increased in acute DIC; normal or slightly increased in chronic DIC
- APTT: activated partial thromboplastin time is increased in acute DIC; normal, sometimes decreased, in chronic DIC
- additional: there is sometimes evidence of microangiopathic haemolytic anaemia – schistocytes; increased serum LDH; decreased serum haptoglobin; common in renal or malignant disease.

Theme: Haemolytic anaemia

150 E: Paroxysmal nocturnal haemoglobinuria
Flow cytometric analysis of red cells has replaced Ham's test. The bone marrow is sometimes hypoplastic, despite haemolysis.

151 F: Pyruvate kinase deficiency
Pyruvate kinase deficiency (PKD) is one of the most common enzymatic defects of the erythrocyte. The clinical severity of this disorder varies widely, ranging from a mildly compensated anaemia to severe anaemia of childhood. Most individuals who

are affected do not require treatment. PKD is an erythrocyte enzymopathy involving the Embden–Meyerhof pathway of anaerobic glycolysis. Pyruvate kinase (PK) catalyses the conversion of phosphoenolpyruvate to pyruvate. This is one of two glycolytic reactions in the erythrocyte that results in the production of ATP. A discrepancy between erythrocyte energy requirements and ATP-generating capacity produces irreversible membrane injury, resulting in cellular distortion, rigidity and dehydration. This leads to premature erythrocyte destruction by the spleen and liver.

152   G: Sickle cell anaemia

Normal haemoglobin comprises two α and two β chains. In sickle cell disease valine is substituted for glutamic acid at position 6 on the β chain. This single amino acid substitution results in HbS, which is less soluble than HbA – the normal adult form of haemoglobin. The sickle haemoglobin gene is inherited as an autosomal recessive characteristic and is commonly seen in patients of Afro-Caribbean descent. Sickle cell anaemia occurs in homozygotes, whereas the sickle cell trait occurs in heterozygotes. When deoxygenated haemoglobin undergoes polymerisation it produces the characteristic sickle cells.

153   B: Hereditary spherocytosis

Osmotic fragility test is positive. The spleen should be removed in all but the mildest cases.

Theme: Treatment of epilepsy

154   F: Lamotrigine

Lamotrigine is an antiepileptic drug prescribed to treat partial seizures and primary and secondary generalised tonic-clonic seizures. It is also used to treat myoclonic seizures and may be tried for atypical absence, atonic and tonic seizures in patients with the Lennox–Gastaut syndrome. Lamotrigine may cause a serious skin rash, especially in children: dose recommendations should be adhered to closely.

Lamotrigine is used either as sole treatment or as an adjunct to treatment with other antiepileptic drugs. Sodium valproate increases the lamotrigine plasma concentration, whereas the enzyme-inducing antiepileptics reduce it: care is therefore required in choosing the appropriate initial dose and subsequent titration. Where the potential for interaction is unknown, treatment should be initiated with lower doses, such as those used with valproate.

155 I: Sodium valproate

Hepatic enzyme-inducing antiepileptic drugs increase the metabolism of both progesterone and oestrogen. As the concentrations of these hormones may be lowered by 50% or more, adjustments are required in contraceptive regimes to ensure that pregnancy is prevented. Sodium valproate does not interfere with the oestrogen component of the contraceptive pill, unlike phenytoin and carbamazepine.

156 D: Ethosuximide

Although its mechanism of action is uncertain, ethosuximide is thought to work by blocking T-type voltage-gated Ca^{2+} channels in thalamic neurones: these channels are important for the generation of rhythmic activity in the neurones. Ethosuximide is not useful in the treatment of tonic-clonic seizures, but is used as a second-line therapeutic agent for absence seizures.

157 B: Clobazam

Clobazam (CLB) is a new antiepileptic drug and the first 1,5-benzodiazepine (BZP). It has selectivity for the omega-2 receptor, which contributes to its anticonvulsive actions. In contrast, omega-1 receptors are responsible for other CNS activities, such as sedation. CLB has been used as an adjunctive treatment in patients with refractory epilepsies. From both experimental and clinical observations, CLB has been proved to possess a wide spectrum of activity, high effectiveness and good tolerability in several types of epilepsies.

Medicine SBAs

1 A 45-year-old woman presented to the skin clinic with some flaccid blisters involving the front part of her chest: some areas were red and weeping. The dermatologist took a skin biopsy, the results of which show a superficial intraepidermal split just above the basal layer with acantholysis.

What is the SINGLE most likely diagnosis?

A   Bullous pemphigoid   D   Pemphigus vulgaris
B   Dermatitis herpetiformis   E   Tuberous sclerosis
C   Epidermolysis bullosa   ☐

2 A 56-year-old man presents with pinkish-red scaly plaques on the extensor surface of his knees and elbows. The lesions are itchy and sore.

What would be the best SINGLE first-line treatment for this condition?

A   Calcipotriol   D   Phototherapy (UVB and UVA)
B   Dithranol   E   Topical steroids
C   Oral steroids   ☐

3 A 62-year-old politician was finding it increasingly difficult to remember all the information at his daily Party meetings. This was followed by a decline in language function: he found it difficult to remember the names of his colleagues, and planning, organising and abstracting also became difficult. Now, at times, he becomes agitated and aggressive. There is a similar family history.

What is the SINGLE most likely diagnosis?

A   Alzheimer's disease   D   Multi-infarct dementia
B   Creutzfeldt–Jakob disease   E   Parkinson's disease
C   Lewy body dementia   ☐

4 A 24-year-old woman presents with a sudden-onset, severe headache with retro-orbital pain and photophobia, associated with two episodes of vomiting. She says it is the worst headache she has ever had. There is no past history of migraine. Examination reveals no neurological deficit.

What is the SINGLE most appropriate initial investigation?

A   CT scan of the head   D   MRI of the head
B   ESR   E   Technetium brain scan
C   Lumbar puncture

5 A 46-year-old woman presented with persistent morning headaches and vomiting. A CT scan shows a space-occupying lesion in the temporal lobe. Assessment of her visual fields reveals a defect.

What is the SINGLE most likely defect?

A   Bitemporal hemianopia   D   Homonymous upper quadrantic
B   Homonymous hemianopia   defect
C   Homonymous lower   E   Unilateral visual loss
    quadrantic defect

6 A 56-year-old man, with a positive family history of heart problems, has been given a diagnosis of ischaemic heart disease. His cholesterol level is 6.5 mmol/l. He has been started on a statin and given appropriate dietary advice.

Which SINGLE dietary change advice is most likely to increase his cholesterol level?

A   Increase his intake of foods such as pulses, legumes, root vegetables and unprocessed cereals
B   Increase the amount of plant stanol in his diet tenfold by using a margarine containing an added stanol ester, which lowers LDL cholesterol
C   Reduce his intake of dairy products and meat
D   Substitute polyunsaturated for saturated fats in cooking
E   Tell him he can eat modest amounts of eggs and prawns

7 A 32-year-old man diagnosed to have insulin-dependent diabetes mellitus was started on Mixtard® insulin. However, control proved to be a problem, with hypoglycaemia between meals and particularly at night. This was substituted with rapid-acting insulin analogues, but this has resulted in erratic morning blood sugar readings.

What would be the SINGLE best management to overcome this problem?

A   Add in a sulphonylurea
B   Add in the new class of insulin secretagogues – repaglinide
C   Adjust the dose of a rapid-acting insulin according to blood glucose results
D   Use a long-acting insulin analogue
E   Use insulin glargine

8 A 45-year-old smoker of 20 pack-years has incidentally been found on X-ray to have a tumour in his right lung.

Which of the following statements about investigation of this condition is not true?

A   Bilateral lymphangitis carcinomatosa on chest X-ray is more often indicative of a primary tumour in the lung
B   Breath scan has about 85% specificity in predicting lung cancer without histology
C   CT-guided fine-needle aspiration is associated with pneumothorax in 25% of cases
D   MRI is more effective than a CT scan in the staging of lung cancer
E   Spirometry, especially FEV_1, is a must to decide the appropriateness of surgery

9 A 45-year-old man presented to his doctor with gradually
progressive shortness of breath. His GP requested a chest X-ray,
which shows bilateral interstitial opacities.

*The following facts about differential diagnosis of his condition are
true, except:*

A A history of working in the aerospace industry, together with chest
X-ray features of bilateral interstitial opacities would indicate a
diagnosis of berylliosis

B A prolonged history of therapy with non-steroidal
anti-inflammatory drugs (NSAIDs) for background rheumatoid
arthritis would help in explaining the condition

C Crocidolite is the most likely type of asbestos to produce
asbestosis and mesothelioma

D Gross clubbing with bilateral interstitial opacities could indicate
usual interstitial pneumonia of Liebow

E If this man were a farmer by profession, then diurnal variation of
symptoms and fever, tachypnoea and coarse inspiratory
crackles on examination would give us the diagnosis   ☐

10 A 52-year-old man presented with recurrent episodes of malaise
with cough, breathlessness and fever. A chest X-ray showed a
confluent patchy parenchymal shadowing; lung function testing
revealed a restrictive defect. His ESR was raised. An open lung
biopsy shows characteristic buds of connective tissue.

What is the SINGLE most likely diagnosis?

A Bronchiolitis obliterans with organising pneumonia
B Goodpasture's syndrome
C Kaposi's sarcoma
D *Pneumocystis jiroveci* pneumonia (new name for *Pneumocystis
carinii*)
E Pneumonia due to *Mycobacterium avium intracellulare*   ☐

11 A 52-year-old man had been visiting his GP for a long time, complaining of low backache. He also suffered from deafness in his right ear and used a hearing aid. After being on NSAIDs for 2 years, he presented to the hospital with sudden-onset shortness of breath and has been given a diagnosis of heart failure. An X-ray of his lower back shows predominantly lytic lesions and routine blood tests reveal an increased serum alkaline phosphatase level.

What would be the SINGLE most likely treatment strategy for this condition?

A   Calcitonin, sc   D   Pamidronate, iv
B   Calcitriol   E   Raloxifine   *SERM*
C   Danazol   *EVISTA*

12 A 68-year-old woman presented to her GP with general symptoms of tiredness, weight loss and sweating during the night. She was found to be generally depressed. Further enquiry reveals she has stiffness and pain in her shoulders and neck, which is worse in the morning and lasts about 30 minutes.

What is the SINGLE best investigation of choice for this condition?

A   Autoantibody screen   D   Nerve conduction velocity
B   ESR   E   Temporal artery biopsy
C   Muscle biopsy   *GCA*

13 A 33-year-old married man was visiting Thailand with his family when he developed diarrhoea that lasted for 1 week. He returned to the UK and a couple of weeks later presented to his GP complaining of pain in his knee and both heels. His eyes have become red and he has developed some painless, red, confluent plaques on his hands and feet, which his GP has diagnosed as psoriasis.

What is the SINGLE most likely diagnosis?

A   Ankylosing spondylitis   D   Psoriatic arthritis
B   Enteropathic arthritis   E   Reactive arthritis
C   Gonococcal arthritis   *urethritis*
                                 arthritis
                                 conjunctivitis

14 A 52-year-old man, diagnosed with rheumatoid arthritis, was prescribed NSAIDs. However, due to persistent synovitis he was started on methotrexate and referred for physiotherapy. After 6 weeks there was no improvement. Because there was an increase in morning stiffness and in the acute-phase response, he was put on a combination of methotrexate and sulfasalazine. Again, there was no improvement and he was tried on oral gold.

What is the SINGLE best treatment regime at this stage?

A   Azathioprine
B   Combination of gold plus penicillamine
C   Combination of gold, leflunomide and methotrexate
D   Infliximab plus methotrexate
E   Leflunomide

15 A 62-year-old man with a known history of gallstones presented to A&E with severe pain in his upper abdomen and nausea and vomiting. Physical examination showed upper abdominal tenderness but no other systemic abnormalities. Testing reveals him to be tachycardic, hypotensive and oliguric. Blood tests show a raised white cell count, raised serum urea level and a low serum albumin level. Blood gases show that he is hypoxic.

What is the SINGLE best treatment option to include in his management?

A   Morphine sc delivered through a patient-controlled system and nasojejunal tube feeding
B   Nasogastric suction, iv fluids, no antibiotics and Ryle's tube feeding
C   Nasogastric suction, oxygen therapy, iv antibiotics
D   Oxygen therapy, iv antibiotics, total parenteral nutrition and oral non-steroidal agents
E   Subcutaneous morphine pump, iv antibiotics, iv fluids

16 A 32-year-old pregnant woman presented to her GP with pruritus during the third trimester. Liver biochemistry shows a cholestatic picture.

What is the SINGLE most likely outcome?

A   The condition will not resolve after delivery
B   The fetus will probably be harmed
C   The ingestion of oestrogen-containing oral contraceptive pills will decrease the risk
D   The prognosis for the mother is poor
E   There is a minimal risk of recurrence in subsequent pregnancies

17 A 42-year-old man with cirrhosis of the liver and ascites presented with clinical deterioration. Diagnostic aspiration of the ascites fluid shows a raised neutrophil count in the ascites fluid.

Which of the following statements best fits this scenario?

A   If the patient survives, an oral quinolone should be prescribed daily but it does not prolong survival
B   It is an indication for liver transplantation
C   *Staphylococcus epidermidis* is the commonest infecting organism
D   The prognosis is grave, irrespective of the underlying liver disease
E   There is a high mortality and high recurrence rate

18 A 52-year-old postmenopausal woman presented with general fatigue. A series of blood tests were performed to find the cause. Results show her to have a high serum aminotransferase level and a mild elevation of both ALP and bilirubin. A full blood count shows mild normocytic normochromic anaemia with thrombocytopenia and leucopenia. Liver biopsy shows chronic inflammatory cell infiltrate with lymphocytes, plasma cells and sometimes lymphoid follicles in the portal tracts.

What is the SINGLE most probable diagnosis?

A α_1-AT deficiency
B   Autoimmune hepatitis
C   Chronic hepatitis C infection
D   Infectious mononucleosis
E   Non-alcoholic steatohepatitis (NASH)

19 A 62-year-old woman presents with an acute variceal bleed. ☐

Which of the following management options is evidence-based?

A Intravenous prophylactic antibiotics have not been shown to reduce mortality

B Intravenous vasopressin has not been shown to reduce mortality

C Patients treated on a medical ward do as well as those on a high-dependency, intensive-care nursing unit because of the high risk of ITU nosocomial infection

D Sucralfate is known to reduce oesophageal ulceration when used as a conservative treatment

E Variceal sclerotherapy and banding are temporary measures ☐

20 A 36-year-old man presents with upper abdominal pain. When asked specifically where the pain is, he points to the epigastrium. He says the pain occurs more during the day and is worse when he is hungry, but antacids relieve it. You suspect he has a duodenal ulcer.

Which of the following facts about Helicobacter pylori *is true?*

A *Helicobacter* immunoassay on a stool sample can be used for the qualitative detection of the *H. pylori* antigen, and is useful for monitoring the efficacy of eradication therapy

B Histological examination of tissue biopsy samples (usually four, taken from different parts of the stomach lining) permits detection of the bacterium without evaluation of tissue damage

C IgG antibodies to *H. pylori* can be found in saliva, and are likely to give false-negative results in those who have recently taken antibiotics, bismuth compounds or omeprazole.

D In infected tissues, it takes about 1 day for the changes in the CLO test to become apparent

E The [^{13}C]urea breath test can be used to demonstrate eradication of the organism following treatment ☐

21 A 72-year-old man presented with progressive and unrelenting dysphagia. Initially, he had difficulty swallowing solids but then also had difficulty with liquids. Endoscopy shows an ulcerative lesion extending around the wall of the oesophagus, producing narrowing.

Which of the following applies to the management of such cases?

A   Adenocarcinomas can be treated with radiotherapy

B   5-FU + cisplatin and combined chemo/radiotherapy is being used in some centres and giving some prolongation of survival

C   Although only 10% of tumours are resectable, operative mortality is now less than 40%

D   Patients who present with stage I disease have a 5-year survival rate of 30%

E   Photocoagulation therapy using a laser beam delivered through an endoscope is an effective way of prolonging survival

22 A 26-year-old obese man presents to the clinic. He is found to have a BMI of 36 and wants advice regarding treatment of his obesity.

Which of the following pertains to the treatment of obesity?

A   Fenfluramine has now been banned in the UK because it causes systemic hypertension

B   Orlistat causes weight loss by inhibiting pancreatic and gastric lipase

C   The removal of large amounts of fat by liposuction tends to be quite effective in cases of sudden weight gain

D   Weight loss will be very slow at first when only glycogen breaks down, but this is followed 3–4 weeks later by a period of incremental weight loss due to the breakdown of adipose tissue

E   With morbid obesity at presentation in the under 18-year-old age group, restrictive surgery, which limits the size of the stomach so the person feels full after eating a small amount of food, may sometimes be tried before pharmacotherapy

23 A 46-year-old HIV-positive man, on treatment, developed fever, malaise and anorexia. He also complained of diarrhoea and was found to have malabsorption and anaemia. The organism responsible was isolated on direct examination and culture of a bone marrow sample. He is being treated with a combination of ethambutol, rifabutin and clarithromycin.

What is the SINGLE most likely organism?

A   *Cryptosporidium parvum*
B   *Mycobacterium avium intracellulare*
C   *Mycobacterium tuberculosis*
D   *Pneumocystis jiroveci*
E   *Pseudomonas aeruginosa*

24 A 36-year-old woman is found to have advanced HIV disease.

Strategic planning in antiretroviral use includes which of the following?

A   Intravenous didanosine is used for the treatment of pregnant women
B   Patients should start treatment before their CD4 count drops below 200 cells/ml
C   Patients with a CD4 count between 200 and 350 cells/ml who have a high viral load or a rapidly falling CD4 count, may be considered for early intervention
D   Treatment is with three nucleoside analogues
E   Use of zidovudine in post-exposure prophylaxis for needlestick injuries in healthcare workers is shown to remove the risk of seroconversion

Medicine SBAs – Answers

1   D: Pemphigus vulgaris
This occurs in the middle-aged population and affects both sexes
equally. Rarely, the disease can be drug-induced (eg penicillamine
or angiotensin-converting enzyme (ACE) inhibitors). Treatment
is with very high doses of oral prednisolone.

2   B: Dithranol
Topical dithranol is most likely to induce remission. Psoriasis that
is unresponsive to topical therapy is treated with phototherapy
(UVB and UVA) or systemic therapy (methotrexate, acitretin or
hydroxyurea). Topical steroids and calcipotriol are generally used
as second-line agents.

3   A: Alzheimer's disease
People particularly at risk of developing Alzheimer's disease are
those with a family history of the disease, those who have
sustained a head injury or those who have Down's syndrome.
Neuropathological changes include neuronal reduction,
neurofibrillary tangles, senile neurotic plaques and a variable
amyloid angiopathy. Aggregation of amyloid appears to be a
central event. The gene for the amyloid precursor protein (*APP*) is
localised close to the defect on chromosome 21. Dementia is
diagnosed clinically from the patient's history and examination,
especially cognitive testing, but it can also be confirmed by
psychometric testing.

4   A: CT scan of the head
CT imaging is the initial investigation of choice, which usually
shows the presence of subarachnoid or intraventricular blood. A
lumbar puncture is unnecessary if a subarachnoid haemorrhage is
confirmed by CT, but should be considered if doubt remains. The
CSF becomes yellow (xanthochromic) about 12 hours after a
subarachnoid haemorrhage. MRI angiography is usually
performed in all patients who are potentially fit for surgery.

5   D: Homonymous upper quadrantic defect
Temporal lobe lesions cause an upper quadrantic defect and
parietal lobes a lower one. A lesion to the optic chiasma causes

bitemporal hemianopia. Optic tract lesions cause field defects, which are homonymous, hemianopic and often incomplete and incongruous.

6   D: Substitute polyunsaturated fats for saturated fats in cooking

Monosaturated oils, particularly olive oil and polyunsaturated oils like sunflower oil, safflower oil and soya oil, should be used in cooking. Currently, it is believed that around 42% of the energy in the typical British diet comes from fat. Dietary advice is to reduce this percentage. The COMA (Committee on Medical Aspects of Food Policy) report advocated that no more than 35% of the daily energy requirement should come from fat, while the NACNE (National Advisory Committee on Nutritional Education) paper recommends a reduction to no more than 30%. Special emphasis is placed on reducing the amount of saturated fat in the diet.

7   E: Use insulin glargine

Insulin glargine has a modified structure to reduce its solubility, thus prolonging its duration of action. Therefore it has a less peaked concentration profile in the blood than conventional long-acting insulins.

8   A: Bilateral lymphangitis carcinomatosa on chest X-ray is more often indicative of a primary tumour in the lung

Bilateral lymphangitis carcinomatosa is more often associated with infradiaphragmatic primaries, eg stomach and colon.

9   B: A prolonged history of therapy with NSAIDs could be responsible

Therapy with agents such as amiodarone, hexamethonium, nitrofurantoin, paraquat, continuous oxygen and cytotoxic agents can lead to diffuse lung injury, infiltrates and/or fibrosis. Exposure to NSAIDs generally results in asthma, with or without rhinitis.

10   A: Bronchiolitis obliterans with organising pneumonia

No causative infective agent has been described and the disease is of unknown aetiology. The diagnosis is usually made on the history and X-ray appearances. Although there is a dramatic response to corticosteroid therapy, the disease recurs episodically.

11   D: Pamidronate, iv

Although intravenous pamidronate is highly efficacious, it can be associated with first-dose reactions characterised by flu-like symptoms, including transient pyrexia over 24–48 hours. In trials lasting for up to 18 months, a 50–70% reduction in serum alkaline phosphatase levels was seen in over 80% of the patients treated with oral bisphosphonates, eg tiludronate and alendronate.

12   B: ESR

Polymyalgia rheumatica is characterised by raised ESR and C-reactive protein (CRP) levels. The diagnosis should be questioned if these levels are not raised. Serum alkaline phosphatase and gamma-glutamyl transferase (GGT) may also be elevated. A temporal artery biopsy shows giant-cell arthritis in about 10–30% of cases, but is not usually performed.

13   E: Reactive arthritis

A variety of organisms can trigger reactive arthritis. It is typically an acute, asymmetrical, lower limb arthritis, occurring a few days to a couple of weeks after infection. Sacroiliitis and spondylitis may develop. Acute anterior uveitis may complicate more severe disease. The skin lesions resemble psoriasis (circinate balanitis and keratoderma blenorrhagica). The classic triad of Reiter's disease is urethritis, arthritis and conjunctivitis.

14   D: Infliximab plus methotrexate

Infliximab is a monoclonal antibody directed against tumour necrosis factor-alpha (TNF-α) and is given iv. Infliximab is co-prescribed with methotrexate to prevent a loss of efficacy because of antibody formation. Both products halt bone erosion in up to 70% of patients with rheumatoid arthritis (RA) and produce healing in a few. As a side-effect, some people become autoantibody-positive and develop a reversible lupus-like syndrome. Reactivation of old TB may occur.

15   A: Morphine sc delivered through a patient-controlled system and nasojejunal tube feeding

Instigation of total parenteral nutrition has been associated with a high risk of infection. Nasojejunal tube feeding is well tolerated and can maintain adequate nutritional input. Some patients will require positive-pressure ventilation and often renal support. The mortality rate for this last group of patients, however, is extremely high.

16   B: The fetus will probably be harmed

Intrahepatic cholestasis of pregnancy is associated with increased fetal loss. Recurrent cholecystitis may occur during subsequent pregnancies.

17   E: There is a high mortality and a high recurrence rate

This is one of the most serious complications of ascites and occurs in approximately 8% of cases of cirrhosis with ascites. The infecting organisms gain access to the peritoneum by haematogenous spread. Features of chest pain and pyrexia are frequently absent. The condition has a 25% mortality rate and recurs in 70% of patients within a year.

18   B: Autoimmune hepatitis

There are two peaks according to age in the presentation. Patients in the perimenopausal age group present with non-specific symptoms, whereas patients in the teenage and early twenties age group present with an acute hepatitis and with jaundice and higher aminotransferase levels, which do not improve with time. Three types of autoimmune hepatitis have been recognised: type I with antibodies (antinuclear, anti-smooth muscle); type II with antibodies (anti-LKM1); and type III with soluble liver antigen. Type II mostly occurs in girls and young women. Again, there are two types of liver-kidney microsomal antibodies: type 2 is found in other autoimmune diseases.

19   B: Intravenous vasopressin has not been shown to reduce mortality

Sucralfate is known to reduce oesophageal ulceration following endoscopic therapy. Intravenous prophylactic antibiotics reduce infections. The only vasoconstrictor that has been shown to reduce the mortality rate is terlipressin. It should not be given to patients with ischaemic heart disease; the patient will complain of abdominal colic, will defecate and will have facial pallor due to generalised vasoconstriction.

20   E: The [^{13}C]urea breath test can be used to demonstrate eradication of the organism following treatment

Patients infected with *Helicobacter pylori* have immunoglobulin antibodies to the organism. Tests for the detection of antibodies to *H. pylori* circulating in the blood, or found in the saliva, have excellent sensitivity and specificity of over 95%, and are cheap and simple compared with invasive techniques. They can give very quick results, even within minutes of the first consultation, and are the only tests that are not likely to give false-negative results in patients who have recently taken antibiotics, bismuth compounds or omeprazole (NIH Consensus Conference, 1994). Immunoassay in stool can only be used for qualitative detection. Histological examination of tissue biopsy samples (usually four, taken from different parts of the stomach lining) permits detection of the bacterium together with evaluation of tissue damage. Most cases of infection can be detected with a haematoxylin & eosin (H&E) stain of gastric tissue, but special stains like Giemsa can be used if H&E results are inconclusive. In infected tissues the change occurs within about 1 hour, so that the results of the CLO test are often available while the patient is still in the endoscopy unit, meaning that therapy decisions can be made immediately.

21   B: 5-FU + cisplatin and combined chemo/radiotherapy is being used in some centres and giving some prolongation of survival

Adenocarcinomas are not radiosensitive and surgery is the mainstay of treatment, whereas squamous-cell carcinomas can be treated with either surgery or radiotherapy. However, only 40% tumours are resectable but the operative mortality is now less than 10%. For surgery, a 10-cm proximal clearance is needed to avoid submucosal spread. Various surgical procedures can be used: total gastrectomy, carried out via the thoracoabdominal approach (adenocarcinoma); a subtotal, two-stage oesophagectomy (Ivor Lewis); a subtotal, three-stage oesophagectomy (McKeown); and a trans-hiatal oesophagectomy. Laser therapy produces good palliation in over 60% of cases but may need to be repeated every 4–6 weeks. It is associated with oesophageal perforation in about 5% cases.

22   B: Orlistat causes weight loss by inhibiting pancreatic and
gastric lipase

For the purposes of the NICE guidance, people are considered to
be morbidly obese if they have a body mass index (BMI) of 40
kg/m² or more, or if they have a BMI between 35 kg/m² and 40
kg/m² and other significant disease (for example, diabetes, high
blood pressure) that may be improved if they lose weight. Weight
loss is always greater at first and then slows down significantly.
Surgery is contraindicated in children below the age of 18 years
according to NICE guidelines. NICE has recommended that
surgery should be available as a treatment option provided that
patients meet all of the following criteria:

- They are aged 18 years or over.
- They have been receiving treatment in a specialist obesity clinic
  at a hospital.
- They have tried all other appropriate non-surgical treatments to
  lose weight but have not been able to maintain weight loss.
- There are no specific medical or psychological reasons why they
  should not have this type of surgery.
- They are generally fit enough for an anaesthetic and surgery.
- They should understand that they will need to be followed-up
  by a doctor and other healthcare professionals such as
  dieticians or psychologists over the long term.

There are two main types of surgery available to aid weight loss,
known as 'malabsorptive' and 'restrictive' procedures.
Malabsorptive surgery works by shortening the length of the
digestive tract (gut) so that the amount of food absorbed by the
body is reduced. This type of surgery involves creating a bypass by
joining one part of the intestine to another. Restrictive surgery
limits the size of the stomach so the person feels full after eating a
small amount of food. This type of surgery can involve 'stapling'
parts of the stomach together or fitting a tight band to make a
small pouch for food to enter.

Fenfluramine causes systemic hypertension, which is why it has
been banned.

23   B: *Mycobacterium avium intracellulare (MAI)*
This is typically resistant to standard antituberculous therapies,

although ethambutol may be useful. Primary prophylaxis with rifabutin or azithromycin may delay the appearance of MAI, but no corresponding increase in survival has been shown.
(*Pneumocystis jiroveci* is the new name for *Pneumocystis carinii*.)

24 **C: Patients with a CD4 count between 200 and 350 cells/ml who have a high viral load or a rapidly falling CD4 count, may be considered for early intervention**

Patients should be started on treatment:

- if they have symptomatic HIV disease
- if they have rapidly falling CD4 counts
- if before their CD4 count falls below 200 cells/ml
- if they have a high viral load.

Treatment is with three drugs, two nucleoside analogues in combination with either a non-nucleoside reverse transcriptase inhibitor, a protease inhibitor or abacavir as a third nucleoside analogue. The use of zidovudine has been shown to reduce, but not remove, the risk of seroconversion in healthcare workers. Intravenous zidovudine should be given during labour and zidovudine syrup given to the neonate for the first 6 weeks of life.

Surgery

Acute Surgical Emergencies : General Surgery :
ENT : Ophthalmology : Orthopaedics

Chapter contributed by
Shafiul A. Chowdhury MBBS MRCSI MRCS (Glas.)

Surgery EMQs

Theme: **Epigastric pain**

Options

A   Acute cholecystitis
B   Acute pancreatitis
C   Benign gastric ulcer
D   Biliary colic
E   Chronic pancreatitis

F   Gastric carcinoma
G   Oesophageal varices
H   Oesophagitis
I   Zollinger–Ellison syndrome

Instructions

For each of the patients described below choose the SINGLE most appropriate diagnosis from the list of options above. Each option may be used once, more than once or not at all.

1   A 41-year-old woman presents to A&E with a 2-day history of epigastric pain which is worse after eating fatty foods. Murphy's sign is positive on examination. ☐

2   A 53-year-old man presents in A&E with severe epigastric pain radiating to his back, but says he finds some relief by leaning forwards. He suddenly becomes hypotensive with shortness of breath and is taken to the resuscitation area. This man also has an alcohol problem ☐

3   A 57-year-old man presents with loss of appetite, weight loss and occasional epigastric pain that has recently become worse and more frequent. He is known to have stomach problems, which are managed with antacids. He is a heavy smoker. ☐

4   A 33-year-old man presented with epigastric pain after a heavy meal. His blood parameters were normal and he was apyrexial. The pain has settled with analgesia and he has had no nausea or vomiting. ☐

5   A 78-year-old man admitted by the medical team has been on antibiotics to treat a chest infection. A week later and he is complaining of dysphagia. ☐

Theme: **Initial management of chest trauma**

Options

A	Aortogram	F	MRI
B	Chest drain	G	Oral analgesia
C	CT chest	H	PCA
D	CXR	I	Thoracotomy
E	Lung function tests	J	Ventilation

Instructions

For each of the patients described below choose the SINGLE most appropriate management from the list of options above. Each option may be used once, more than once or not at all.

6 A 70-year-old man fell down the stairs and hit the side of his chest on the floor. His right lower ribs are exquisitely tender. ☐

7 A 16-year-old boy was playing rugby when he was kicked in the chest. Although he initially felt alright, he suddenly now feels unwell, with breathlessness. ☐

8 A 75-year-old woman with a history of falls, injures her back and sustains a fracture in a lumbar transverse process. ☐

9 A 31-year-old man involved in a high-speed RTA has bilateral chest drains inserted. These have started draining at 200 ml/min. ☐

10 A 20-year-old man, planned for operative fracture management, also sustained a chest injury causing a small apical pneumothorax. ☐

Theme: **Incontinence**

Options

A	Anticholinergic drugs	G	Laxative
B	Clean, self-intermittent catheterisation	H	Pelvic floor exercises
		I	Prophylactic antibiotics
C	Desmopressin	J	Tricyclic antidepressant
D	Fluid restriction	K	Vaginal oestrogen
E	Hormones	L	Weight loss
F	Incontinence pants		

Instructions

For each of the patients described below choose the SINGLE most appropriate management from the list of options above. Each option may be used once, more than once or not at all.

11 An 18-year-old woman attempted suicide by jumping from a three-storey building. This has resulted in her having an amputation, a colostomy and long-term catheterisation because of incontinence as she developed an atonic bladder with recurrent infections.

12 A 15-year-old girl recently noticed that her underpants were damp at the end of the day. She has also noticed that she leaks when laughing or coughing. A cystometrogram confirms stress incontinence.

13 A 52-year-old woman has a BMI of 33 and complains of leaks on exertion. Cystometrogram confirms stress incontinence.

14 An 82-year-old man presents with frequency and occasional incontinence. He has some bladder outflow problems but they are not causing him that much bother. He always has a cup of herbal tea before going to bed.

15 A 72-year-old man had a radical prostatectomy a few months ago and now suffers from mild incontinence.

Theme: **Diagnosis of breast disease**

Options

A	Benign breast change	G	Fibroadenoma
B	Carcinoma	H	Mammary duct fistula
C	Cyclical mastalgia	I	Nipple eczema
D	Cyst	J	Non-cyclical mastalgia
E	Duct ectasia	K	Paget's disease
F	Duct papilloma	L	Periductal mastitis

Instructions

For each of the patients described below choose the SINGLE most appropriate diagnosis from the list of options above. Each option may be used once, more than once or not at all.

16 A 55-year-old woman discovered a lump in her right breast 2 months ago. It is firm and irregular and in the upper and outer aspect of the breast. A small palpable lymph node has been found in the left axilla on examination. The supraclavicular nodes are not involved. ☐

17 A 46-year-old woman gives a history of a creamy-green discharge from her right nipple, which is occasionally bloodstained. She has subsequently developed a tender breast lump on the same side. On examination there is a firm lump beneath the areola with surrounding redness. ☐

18 A 24-year-old woman presents with a non-tender lump in her left breast. It is 2.5 cm in diameter, firm, well circumscribed and slips easily between the fingers on testing for fluctuation. ☐

19 A 64-year-old woman develops gradual-onset eczema with a slight lumpy feeling beneath the nipple on the right side. It is not itchy. ☐

20 A 56-year-old woman notices bilateral weepy and pruritic lesions on and around her nipples and areolas. ☐

Theme: **Sudden visual loss**

Options

A	Acute glaucoma	F	Optic neuropathy
B	Cataract	G	PMR
C	Central retinal vein thrombosis	H	Temporal arteritis
D	Chronic simple glaucoma	I	TIA
E	Occlusion of the central retinal artery	J	Uveitis
		K	Vitreous haemorrhage

Instructions

For each of the patients described below choose the SINGLE most appropriate diagnosis from the list of options above. Each option may be used once, more than once or not at all.

21 A 78-year-old man presents with a painful scalp on combing his hair, and with a recent history of uniocular loss of vision. ☐

22 A 58-year-old diabetic presents with sudden visual loss. The red reflex is absent and his retina is difficult to visualise on fundoscopy. ☐

23 A 72-year-old man, who is hypertensive, presents with a sudden loss of vision, which he describes as like a 'curtain coming down'. ☐

24 A 16-year-old girl presents with a transient sudden visual loss. Fundoscopy is normal. ☐

25 A 26-year-old man presents with painful red eyes with a transient loss of vision. ☐

Theme: **Epistaxis**

Options

A   Anticoagulant overdose
B   Coagulopathy
C   Hypertension
D   Local infection
E   Maxillary antral carcinoma
F   Nasal polyps
G   Nasopharyngeal carcinoma
H   Orf
I   Septal perforation

Instructions

For each of the patients described below choose the SINGLE most appropriate diagnosis from the list of options above. Each option may be used once, more than once or not at all.

26 A 69-year-old man with a history of an artificial heart-valve operation presents with epistaxis. ☐

27 A 49-year-old furniture worker presents with anaesthesia of his left cheek and epistaxis. ☐

28 A 56-year-old man who works in a chrome-plating factory presents with recurrent epistaxis. On examination, forceful breathing through his nose produces a whistling effect. ☐

29 A 47-year-old sheep farmer gives a history of epistaxis. Examination reveals a bleeding nasal polyp. ☐

30 A 70-year-old man comes to A&E with epistaxis that has been going on for the last 90 minutes. He is unable to tell you what medication he is taking. However, he does tell you that his pills ran out, but, because he was feeling unwell, he couldn't go and get some more from the chemist. ☐

Theme: **Aortic aneurysm**

Options

A	Abdominal USS	F	Plain AXR
B	Coronary angiogram	G	Resuscitate and immediate
C	CXR		transfer to theatre
D	Echo	H	Spiral CT
E	Lower limb angiogram		

Instructions

For each of the patients described below choose the SINGLE most appropriate management from the list of options above. Each option may be used once, more than once or not at all.

31 A 72-year-old man with known hypertension may have an aortic aneurysm. This diagnosis needs to be excluded. ☐

32 A 63-year-old man is planned for elective AAA repair: its extent and its relationship to the renal arteries need to be identified. ☐

33 A 65-year-old man presents with sudden-onset abdominal pain radiating to his back. He is in shock and has a palpable, tender epigastric mass. ☐

34 A 68-year-old man with known AAA presents with chest pain. ECG reveals unstable angina. ☐

35 A 72-year-old man with a known aortic aneurysm is scheduled to undergo resection of his urinary bladder under general anaesthesia. ☐

Theme: **Thyroid neoplasia**

Options

A   Adenoma
B   Anaplastic
C   Follicular

D   Lymphoma
E   Medullary
F   Papillary

Instructions

For each of the descriptions below choose the SINGLE most appropriate diagnosis from the list of options above. Each option may be used once, more than once or not at all.

36 This has a bad prognosis. ☐

37 Spreads mainly via blood. ☐

38 Has a relationship with MEN. ☐

39 It is difficult to discern whether or not this is malignant by FNAC. ☐

40 Occurs in the iodine-rich areas of the thyroid gland. ☐

Theme: **Investigation of UTI**

Options

A	Creatinine clearance	F	MSU
B	CT	G	Urodynamics
C	Cystoscopy	H	Uroflow
D	Isotope scanning	I	USS KUB
E	Micturating cystourethrogram		

Instructions

For each of the patients described below choose the SINGLE most appropriate investigation from the list of options above. Each option may be used once, more than once or not at all.

41 A 64-year-old man presents with lower urinary tract symptoms. Examination reveals an enlarged prostate. ☐

42 A 3-year-old boy presents with a positive growth of organisms in an MSU.

43 A 48-year-old woman presents with recurrent UTI. USS KUB is normal. ☐

44 A 53-year-old woman with recurrent UTIs complains of haematuria. She smokes 20 cigarettes a day. ☐

45 A 16-year-old girl presents with a continuous burning sensation on passing urine. Her GP tried her on some empirical antibiotics but there was no response. ☐

Theme: **Hip problems**

Options

A Congenital dysplasia of the   D Perthes disease
   hip (CDH)   E Septic arthritis
B Fracture of the hip   F Slipped upper femoral
C Osteoarthritis (OA) of the hip   epiphysis (SUFE)

painless limp

Instructions

For each of the patients described below choose the SINGLE most appropriate diagnosis from the list of options above. Each option may be used once, more than once or not at all.

46 A 2-year-old girl presents with limping due to shortening of her right leg. Examination reveals that the leg is not tender. There are asymmetrical groin creases where the hip does not abduct fully. The Trendelenburg test is positive. ☐

47 A 12-year-old, obese boy presents limping, with pain in his right groin. Examination reveals limitation in flexion, abduction and medial rotation. ☐

48 A 4-year-old boy presents with a limp and restricted movements of his left hip. X-ray of the left hip shows widening of the joint spaces. ☐

49 A 78-year-old woman presents with a gradual reduction in mobility and increasing pain in her hips on movement. She needs to use a walking stick now. ☐

50 A 92-year-old man is brought to A&E having fallen off his bed. He is unable to stand. On examination his left leg is found to be shortened and externally rotated. ☐

Theme: **Accidental injuries in children**

Options

A   Clavicle fracture

B   Greenstick fracture

C   NAI

D   Pulled elbow

E   Scaphoid fracture

F   Supracondylar fracture

Instructions

For each of the patients described below choose the SINGLE most appropriate diagnosis from the list of options above. Each option may be used once, more than once or not at all.

51 A 5-year-old girl slipped and twisted her right elbow while holding her father's hand.

52 A 10-year-old boy fell from a tree and injured his right elbow. It is very swollen and the radial pulse is absent.

53 A 3-month-old baby rolled off the bed and has sustained multiple injuries.

54 A 12-year-old boy fell off a 1.8 m (6 ft) wall trying to imitate a 'super hero' and has injured his left shoulder. He is in immense pain and is unable to lift his shoulder. He is supporting his left elbow with his right hand.

55 A 13-year-old boy fell on his outstretched right hand while playing basketball. He has a tender anatomical snuffbox.

Theme: **Acute abdominal pain in young women**

Options

A   Acute appendicitis
B   Acute cholecystitis
C   Constipation
D   Gastroenteritis
E   Pancreatitis
F   Perforated PU

G   Pneumonia
H   Pyelonephritis
I   Ruptured ectopic pregnancy
J   Ureteric colic
K   UTI

Instructions

For each of the patients described below choose the SINGLE most appropriate diagnosis from the list of options above. Each option may be used once, more than once or not at all.

56 An 18-year-old woman presented with lower abdominal pain, urinary frequency and dysuria. She is pyrexial and has right iliac fossa and rebound tenderness.

57 A 23-year-old woman presents with sudden-onset lower abdominal pain that came on 4 hours ago. She is rolling in agony. She has right iliac fossa and rebound tenderness. A pregnancy test is positive.

58 A 27-year-old heavy smoker with a history of indigestion presents to A&E with generalised abdominal pain. She is found to be in shock and is lying very still on the examination couch.

59 A 33-year-old woman presents with severe epigastric pain that came on after she had her dinner. Murphy's sign is positive.

60 A 24-year-old woman complains of a left-sided loin to groin pain. She is pyrexial and had rigors the previous night. Dipstick urinalysis is positive for blood.

Theme: **Urological disorders**

Options

A	Renal angiomyolipoma	E	Transitional-cell carcinoma
B	Renal-cell carcinoma		of the urinary bladder
C	Retroperitoneal fibrosis	F	Ureteric calculus
D	Transitional-cell carcinoma		
	of the ureter		

Instructions

For each of the patients described below choose the SINGLE most appropriate diagnosis from the list of options above. Each option may be used once, more than once or not at all.

61 A 60-year-old smoker presented with painless haematuria. His plain X-ray KUB was normal. An intravenous urogram (IVU) shows a dilated right pelvicaliceal system up to the level of the vesico-ureteric junction where there is an irregular filling defect in the urinary bladder. ☐

62 A 74-year-old woman came to A&E with a history of hypotension, left abdominal pain and a mass in the left hypochondrium. The patient was resuscitated and responded effectively. Once the patient was stable she underwent a CT scan which has revealed a left renal mass with a surrounding haematoma. ☐

63 A 33-year-old man was seen in A&E with an intermittent colicky right loin to groin pain associated with a temperature of 38.0 °C and rigors. Dipstick urinalysis showed a trace of blood. X-ray KUB was normal, but an IVU has revealed a delayed nephrogram on the right side. ☐

64 A 32-year-old man underwent a para-aortic lymph node dissection for testicular cancer. At USS he has been found to have bilateral hydronephrosis. ☐

65 A 56-year-old man presents with right loin pain and haematuria. He recently noticed a lumpy feeling in his left hypochondrium. ☐

Theme: **Sutures**

Options

A   3–0 nylon

B   4–0 nylon

C   5–0 nylon

D   No.1 loop nylon

E   PDS

F   Prolene

G   Silk

H   Staples

I   Vicryl

Instructions

For each of the indications described below choose the SINGLE most appropriate suture from the list of options above. Each option may be used once, more than once or not at all.

66 *En-masse* closure   D ☐

67 Hernia repair   F ☐

68 Facial wounds   C ☐

69 Scalp wounds   A ☐

70 Intradermal skin closure   E ☐

71 Securing drains   G ☐

Theme: **Testicular disorders**

Options

A   Epididymal cysts
B   Epididymo-orchitis
C   Hydrocele
D   Hydrocele of the spermatic
    cord

E   Inguinal hernia
F   Seminoma
G   Testicular torsion
H   Torsion of a hydatid of Morgagni
I   Varicocele

Instructions

For each of the patients described below choose the SINGLE most appropriate diagnosis from the list of options above. Each option may be used once, more than once or not at all.

72 A 47-year-old man presented to A&E with a 5-day history of left testicular pain. It initially started with a dull ache and has gradually become worse, to the extent that he now finds it difficult to walk. He is apyrexial. ☐

73 A 31-year-old man presents to the clinic with a 2-month history of a right testicular lump. This was mildly tender at first, but over the last month has become painless. ☐

74 A 12-year-old boy presents with a 3-hour history of excruciating left testicular pain. It is preventing him from walking properly and he finds it difficult to sit on a chair. ☐

75 A 30-year-old man presents with right scrotal pain that has been present on and off for the last 5 months. He has been visiting the gym for the last year on a regular basis. On examination, you cannot get above the swelling. ☐

76 A 58-year-old man has noticed bilateral testicular swellings, which have been present for the last 12–18 months. On examination you can get above the swellings. ☐

Theme: **Anorectal disorders**

Options

A Anal fissure
B Fistula-in-ano
C Ischiorectal abscess
D Perianal abscess
E Perianal haematoma

F Proctalgia fugax
G Rectal carcinoma
H Rectal prolapse
I Solitary rectal ulcer syndrome
J Thrombosed piles

Instructions

For each of the patients described below choose the SINGLE most appropriate diagnosis from the list of options above. Each option may be used once, more than once or not at all.

77 A 22-year-old mother, who gave birth 4 weeks ago, presents with pain on passing stools, with bleeding. A rectal examination is impossible due to the pain.

78 A 73-year-old man presents with rectal bleeding and tenesmus.

79 A 42-year-old man gives a 4-month history of a mass hanging down on defecation. During the last week the mass seems to have remained outside his body and has become exquisitely painful, preventing him from sitting down properly.

80 A 37-year-old man presents with an excruciatingly painful lump adjacent to his anus, which has grown from a pimple-sized swelling over the last 7 days.

81 A 24-year-old woman with Crohn's disease presents complaining that her undergarments are soiled with faecal material.

Theme: **Vomiting in young children**

Options

A	Duplication of intestine	F	Meconium ileus
B	Gastro-oesophageal reflux	G	Mesenteric adenitis
C	Hypertrophic pyloric stenosis	H	Mid-gut volvulus
D	Intussusception	I	Strangulated inguinal hernia
E	Meckel's diverticulum		

Instructions

For each of the patients described below choose the SINGLE most appropriate diagnosis from the list of options above. Each option may be used once, more than once or not at all.

82 A 6-month-old boy was brought into A&E with a history of periods of sudden high-pitched crying and drawing his legs up towards his abdomen. He has had two episodes of bilious vomiting and rectal bleeding. ☐

83 A 26-month-old girl presents with marked pallor and rectal bleeding, which is bright red in colour, but no history of vomiting. Abdominal examination reveals no remarkable findings. ☐

84 A 6-week-old baby is brought with a history of intermittent bilious vomiting and rectal bleeding. On examination, her abdomen is tender. ☐

85 A 4-week-old boy is brought to hospital with a history of weight loss and non-bilious vomiting over the past week. Abdominal examination reveals a mass in the epigastrium. ☐

86 A 2-year-old boy presents with a sausage-shaped lump in his abdomen. He has recently had a cold. ☐

Theme: **Anatomical landmarks**

Options

A   Apex beat
B   Chest-drain insertion
C   Femoral artery pulse is felt
D   Fundus of the gallbladder
E   McBurney's point
F   Stellate ganglion

G   Superficial inguinal ring
H   Termination of the spinal cord
I   Transpyloric plane
J   Vena caval opening into the
    diaphragm

Instructions

For each of the locations described below choose the SINGLE most appropriate landmark from the list of options above. Each option may be used once, more than once or not at all.

87 L1 level ☐

88 Midpoint between the suprasternal notch and pubic symphysis ☐

89 Tip of the ninth costal cartilage ☐

90 Just above the mid-inguinal point ☐

91 Fifth intercostal space in the anterior axillary line ☐

Theme: **Carcinogens**

Options

A	Aflatoxin	F	Ionising radiation
B	Aniline dyes	G	Nickel
C	Asbestos	H	Polyvinyl chloride
D	Benzene	I	Smoking
E	Chromium	J	UV light

Instructions

For each of the carcinomas described below choose the SINGLE most appropriate carcinogen from the list of options above. Each option may be used once, more than once or not at all.

92 Urothelial tumours ☐

93 Nasopharyngeal carcinoma ☐

94 Mesothelioma ☐

95 Hepatoma ☐

96 Skin cancers ☐

Theme: **Prostate problems**

Options

A   Bone scan
B   Hormone therapy
C   Medical management
D   Prostate-specific antigen
E   Radical prostatectomy

F   Transrectal ultrasound biopsy
    of the prostate
G   TURP
H   Urodynamics
I   Uroflow
J   Watchful waiting

Instructions

For each of the patients described below choose the SINGLE most appropriate management from the list of options above. Each option may be used once, more than once or not at all.

97 A 65-year-old man presents with a 6-month history of lower urinary tract symptoms. Uroflow shows moderate obstruction.

98 A 69-year-old man had a prostatic biopsy because of a raised PSA level. The biopsy showed a low-grade adenocarcinoma of the prostate. His CT and bone scans are normal.

99 A 71-year-old man had a TURP 6 months ago but now complains of incontinence.

100 A 75-year-old man has been found to have advanced prostate cancer but no metastasis.

101 A 78-year-old man went into retention and was found to have an enlarged prostate. He was catheterised. He has failed a trial without a catheter 2 weeks after starting on α-blockers.

Theme: **Ear problems**

Options

A   Acoustic neuroma
B   Acute otitis media
C   Blast injury
D   Glue ear

E   Ototoxicity
F   Petrous bone fracture
G   Wax

Instructions

For each of the patients described below choose the SINGLE most appropriate diagnosis from the list of options above. Each option may be used once, more than once or not at all.

102 A 51-year-old man with poor ear hygiene complains of deafness after taking a shower. ☐

103 A 74-year-old man was given gentamicin following a difficult catheterisation. He complains that he has recently become hard of hearing. ☐

104 A 24-year-old man presents with right earache that has worsened over the last 24 hours. This has now improved, with a purulent discharge from the ear. ☐

105 A 24-year-old man presents with brown patches that have newly appeared on his trunk. ☐

106 A 34-year-old woman was involved in a car RTA. After recovering she notices that she cannot hear on her right side. ☐

Theme: **Jaundiced patients**

Options

A	Acute alcoholic hepatitis	D	Common bile duct stone
B	Carcinoma of the head of the pancreas	E	Gilbert's syndrome
		F	Liver metastasis
C	Charcot's triad (ascending cholangitis)	G	Primary biliary cirrhosis
		H	Primary sclerosing cholangitis

Instructions

For each of the patients described below choose the SINGLE most appropriate diagnosis from the list of options above. Each option may be used once, more than once or not at all.

107 A 34-year-old woman with known inflammatory bowel disease complains of intermittent jaundice, itching, right hypochondriac pain and weight loss. She has a raised alkaline phosphatase level. ☐

108 A 26-year-old man presented with a 4-year history of occasional mild jaundice that became worse during a chest infection. He has moderate unconjugated hyperbilirubinaemia and a liver biopsy is normal. ☐

109 A 51-year-old woman presented with 4-week history of jaundice and weight loss. She has a raised temperature, palmar erythema, spider naevi and hepatomegaly, with mild ascites. The results of blood tests show a raised white cell count and deranged LFTs. ☐

110 A 58-year-old man presents with weight loss, increasing jaundice and epigastric pain. He had an anterior resection of the rectum 4 years ago. He has hepatomegaly with a raised alkaline phosphatase level. ☐

111 A 23-year-old man presents with fever, jaundice and epigastric pain. ☐

Theme: **Dysphagia**

Options

A	Achalasia	E	Impacted food bolus
B	Benign stricture	F	Oesophageal carcinoma
C	Bulbar palsy	G	Oesophageal spasm
D	Globus hystericus	H	Plummer–Vinson syndrome

Instructions

For each of the patients described below choose the SINGLE most appropriate diagnosis from the list of options above. Each option may be used once, more than once or not at all.

112 A 70-year-old man complains of sudden-onset dysphagia during a meal. ☐

113 A 75-year-old man presents with a short history of progressive dysphagia and weight loss. ☐

114 A 27-year-old woman complains of intermittent dysphagia to solids and liquids associated with retrosternal discomfort. ☐

115 A 57-year-old man has a 10-year history of reflux symptoms. He notices that solid foods occasionally stick retrosternally. ☐

116 A 45-year-old woman being investigated for anaemia complains of dysphagia. ☐

Theme: **Appropriate use of blood transfusion**

Options

A   FFP
B   Platelets
C   RBC

D   RBC in additive solution
E   Whole blood

Instructions

For each of the statements below choose the SINGLE most appropriate blood product from the list of options above. Each option may be used once, more than once or not at all.

117 Requires gentle agitation in storage. ☐

118 Patient with ITP going for surgery. ☐

119 Patient needs to go for urgent surgery but has a high INR. ☐

120 Usually requires pooling for collection. ☐

121 Can be stored for up to 4 weeks. ☐

Theme: **Acute trauma life support**

Options

A	Chest-drain insertion	F	Pericardiocentesis
B	ECG	G	Secondary survey
C	Guedel airway	H	Thomas splint
D	Intubation	I	Trauma X-ray series
E	Needle thoracocentesis	J	Two wide-bore cannulas and iv fluids

Instructions

For each of the patients described below choose the SINGLE most appropriate management from the list of options above. Each option may be used once, more than once or not at all.

122 A 20-year-old woman has been brought to the resuscitation room after being involved in a high-speed RTA. Her airway and breathing are clear. She has a raised JVP, hypotension and muffled heart sounds. ☐

123 A 57-year-old man fell from his roof while installing an antenna and landed on his head. His GCS score is 7.

124 A 17-year-old boy is brought to A&E after a motorbike accident in which he injured his right tibia. His airway and breathing are clear and observations are stable. ☐

125 A 34-year-old man presents to A&E following an RTA. His breathing is laboured and you can hear a moaning sound, even after chin lift and jaw thrust. ☐

126 A 54-year-old man presents with cyanosis and breathlessness following an RTA. Chest percussion is hyper-resonant. ☐

Surgery EMQs – Answers

Theme: Epigastric pain

1 A: Acute cholecystitis

The symptoms in this case are classic for acute cholecystitis. So, in every patient presenting with epigastric pain you should keep this diagnosis as a possibility at the back of your mind. You should also remember that many patients cannot always appreciate the difference between epigastric and right hypochondriac pain.

2 B: Acute pancreatitis

Any patient in pain and shock should be managed with the utmost urgency (may even need transfer to the resuscitation unit or ITU) as they can deteriorate very quickly.

3 F: Gastric carcinoma

These patients nearly always have some sort of dyspepsia, which they may fail to mention at the time of presentation. Therefore, patients with gastric ulcers should be looked at carefully whenever they are seen in clinic.

4 D: Biliary colic

When the gallbladder tries to empty its contents against pressure, eg stones, then it produces a colic. When it is inflamed, it becomes cholecystitis.

5 H: Oesophagitis

Candida oesophagitis is seen in such cases, especially in those who are immunocompromised.

Theme: Initial management of chest trauma

6 G: Oral analgesia

If the patient's observations are stable, with a clear chest, then he should receive strong analgesia. But remember CXRs are not indicated in the case of rib fractures.

7   B: Chest drain
Your clinical findings will guide you as to whether it is a pneumo-
or haemothorax (you don't need an X-ray!). Insert the drain
according to findings (ie passing the tube downwards if it is a
haemothorax and upwards if it is a pneumothorax).

8   F: MRI
It is not always possible to appreciate spinal injuries from plain
X-rays, but MRI gives very good views of the actual extent of the
injury.

9   I: Thoracotomy
This means the patient is losing blood very quickly and you need
to arrest further bleeding physically. If your hospital does not have
the facilities, then you need to resuscitate the patient and organise
his safe transfer to a specialised centre.

10   E: Lung function tests
These tests are a good means of assessing whether a patient with
some lung pathology is fit for anaesthesia.

Theme: Incontinence

11   B: Clean, self-intermittent catheterisation
This patient cannot appreciate how her bladder is functioning.
Such cases are managed by training the patient to empty her
bladder at regular intervals during a specified period. A long-term
catheter could be the solution, but can cause recurrent UTIs.

12   H: Pelvic floor exercises
This is a young woman and pelvic floor exercise will strengthen
her pelvic muscles. Any intervention should ideally be preceded
by conservative measures.

13   L: Weight loss
She is obese, and therefore needs to lose weight to reduce the
added pressure on her bladder.

14   D: Fluid restriction

In this case 'fluid restriction' means the restriction or reduction of fluid intake from evening onwards, in order to reduce frequency, especially as a cup of tea before bedtime does increase urinary frequency.

15   F: Incontinence pants

As the incontinence is mild, it will settle in time.

Theme: Diagnosis of breast disease

16   B: Carcinoma

Any breast lump in older women should be treated with the utmost caution, especially when you find palpable lymph nodes. Depending on the stage of the disease, the recommended treatment in the UK varies from lumpectomy, mastectomy, axillary node sampling, axillary node dissection, chemotherapy to hormone therapy.

17   E: Duct ectasia

This occurs around the menopause, when hypertrophy of the duct epithelium causes blocking of the duct and proximal dilatation (ectasia). It may be confused with cancer, especially when an abscess causes the formation of a lump, which may retract the nipple.

18   G: Fibroadenoma

Nicknamed 'breast mouse'. Typically seen in younger women, they carry a very small risk of malignancy. Most are resected for reassurance, but small ones can be left alone.

19   K: Paget's disease

Unilateral eczematous change is suspicious of Paget's disease or malignancy.

20   I: Nipple eczema

Simultaneous bilateral changes would be an unlikely indication of malignancy. Eczema should be the first thought when the symptoms are bilateral and itchy.

Theme: Sudden visual loss

21 H: Temporal arteritis

Inflammation of the temporal artery results in tenderness of the scalp, which responds well to treatment with steroids.

22 K: Vitreous haemorrhage

Commonly seen in diabetics, but it may occur in patients with bleeding disorders, retinal detachment and central retinal vein occlusion.

23 J: Uveitis

Patients who have suffered a TIA experience a temporary loss of vision, termed 'amaurosis fugax', which may proceed to permanent visual loss.

24 F: Optic neuropathy

Normal fundoscopy gives a hint that the pathology lies behind the fundus.

25 J: Uveitis

Painful red eyes are usually due to inflammation.

Theme: Epistaxis

26 A: Anticoagulant overdose

Since this patient has been fitted with an artificial heart valve and will be on anticoagulants, you may have to stop the anticoagulant, check his INR and proceed to nasal packing.

27 E: Maxillary antral carcinoma

Maxillary antral cancers involve the whole of the antral walls, which results in various presentations, including nerve involvement leading to anaesthesia of the cheek.

28 I: Septal perforation

This is due to ischaemia of the septal vasculature. Referral to an ENT specialist is warranted.

29 H: Orf

Orf (synonym: contagious pustular dermatitis) is an infectious disease acquired from sheep and cattle and seen in people involved in this trade.

30   C: Hypertension
Always enquire about past medical problems and medications, which may give a clue to the presentation.

Theme: Aortic aneurysm

31   A: Abdominal USS
An ultrasound scan is a very efficient diagnostic tool for assessing the presence of an aneurysm in the initial stages.

32   H: Spiral CT
A CT scan is required to assess the accurate position of the aneurysm, which will then dictate the plan of operative management.

33   G: Resuscitate and immediate transfer to theatre
No time should be spent assessing this unstable patient and sending him for a CT scan as this is a surgical emergency. In an acute situation like this, the patient should be taken to theatre as soon as possible for a laparotomy.

34   C: CXR
A chest X-ray should performed to rule out other causes of chest pain.

35   D: Echo
This should be done to assess left ventricular (LV) function as a part of the anaesthetic work-up.

Theme: Thyroid neoplasia

36   B: Anaplastic
Anaplastic means poorly differentiated and therefore most obviously has a poor prognosis.

37   C: Follicular
Follicular cancers spread mainly via the circulatory system.

38 E: Medullary

Medullary cancers are related to multiple endocrine neoplasia (MEN) syndromes.

39 C: Follicular

FNAC fails to differentiate between follicular adenoma and carcinoma and therefore the thyroid is removed in both cases.

40 F: Papillary

Papillary cancers mainly occur in iodine-rich areas.

Theme: Investigation of UTI

41 H: Uroflow

Middle-aged men are likely to have enlarged prostates. For this reason they present with bladder outflow-obstruction symptoms and retain urine in their bladders, which is the growth medium for organisms that cause UTIs. Uroflow will objectively ascertain the actual degree of obstruction and dictate further management.

42 E: Micturating cystourethrogram

Any boy with a first episode of a UTI must be treated with caution and investigated for vesico-ureteric reflux and other renal pathology.

43 C: Cystoscopy

In this case ultrasound scanning of the kidneys, ureter and bladder (USS KUB) has excluded renal pathology, and therefore a look into the bladder is warranted to see if there is any other cause for the UTI.

44 C: Cytoscopy

This should be performed to rule out a bladder tumour.

45 F: MSU

A mid-stream urine sample should be sent for culture and sensitivity testing of her UTI to the current and other antibiotics.

Theme: Hip problems

46 **A: Congenital dysplasia of the hip (CDH)**
This is a late presentation. Ortolani's or Barlow's test should successfully screen for this disorder at birth, which resolves spontaneously within 3 weeks. A higher incidence is noted in breech deliveries and in cases of intrauterine malposition.

47 **F: Slipped upper femoral epiphysis (SUFE)**
This affects 10–16-year-old children. If untreated, it results in avascular necrosis or malunion, leading to arthritis.

48 **D: Perthes disease**
Osteochondritis of the femoral head (Perthes disease) affects children between 3 and 11 years of age. Late X-ray changes show a decrease in the size of the femoral head with patchy density. Treatment is bedrest until the pain subsides and X-ray surveillance. Those with a worse prognosis may need surgery.

49 **C: Osteoarthritis (OA) of the hip**
Elderly people with osteoarthritis usually present with joint pain and reduced mobility which is confirmed on X-ray.

50 **B: Fracture of the hip**
Fracture of the hip is the most frequently encountered case in the emergency department. The history of this elderly patient has all the signs pointing to this diagnosis.

Theme: Accidental injuries in children

51 **D: Pulled elbow**
Such swinging and twisting movements result in dislocation, which can be effectively reduced.

52 **F: Supracondylar fracture**
Any elbow injury with loss of the radial pulse warrants urgent orthopaedic involvement.

53 **C: NAI**
A 3-month-old baby is unable to roll itself off the bed, and any multiple injuries (including fractures) in any young child should

give rise to a high index of suspicion of non-accidental injury
(NAI). The paediatric team should be involved in the assessment.

54   A: Clavicle fracture
The history of inability to lift the shoulder raises the possibility
that somewhere down the shoulder girdle something has
disrupted, and clavicle fractures are commonly encountered.

55   E: Scaphoid fracture
The presentation is typical of a scaphoid fracture. It is a clinical
diagnosis as the initial X-rays fail to demonstrate the fracture.

Theme: **Acute abdominal pain in young
              women**

56   A: Acute appendicitis
Any young woman with right iliac fossa tenderness should be
given a pregnancy test to rule out an unexpected ectopic
pregnancy. On the other hand, there is no diagnostic test to rule
out acute appendicitis. Therefore, where the clinical eye is your
only diagnostic tool, you should always think about differential
diagnoses.

57   I: Ruptured ectopic pregnancy
See the answer above.

58   F: Perforated PU
For any patient in shock and lying still, think 'peritonitis', and the
additional history will direct you to the underlying cause.

59   B: Acute cholecystitis
Murphy's sign is a classic sign of acute cholecystitis.

60   J: Ureteric colic
Loin to groin pain is characteristic for ureteric colic.

Theme: Urological disorders

61 E: Transitional-cell carcinoma of the urinary bladder
Here the bladder tumour has involved the right vesico-ureteric junction, or has obstructed the right ureteric orifice.

62 A: Renal angiomyolipoma
In these cases there is usually an association with tuberous sclerosis. Patients present in childhood with a history of epilepsy. However, it may be seen in elderly people as an unusual presentation.

63 F: Ureteric calculus
Any patient with loin to groin pain and with microscopic haematuria on dipstick testing should give rise to a high suspicion of ureteric calculus. Sometimes, however, this is not seen on a plain X-ray of the kidneys, ureters and bladder (KUB).

64 C: Retroperitoneal fibrosis
Surgery in the retroperitonieal space results in fibrosis and in this case it has involved blockage of the ureters, causing hydronephrosis. The patient should be stented to improve renal function and reviewed.

65 B: Renal-cell carcinoma
The history is the presenting triad for renal-cell carcinoma.

Theme: Sutures

66 D: No. 1 loop nylon
En-masse closure usually involves a non-absorbable suture, bearing in mind Jenkin's rule (length of suture:wound length = 4:1).

67 F: Prolene
This strong non-absorbable suture is the choice for hernia repair.

68 C: 5-0 nylon
Fine sutures are used for facial wounds as there is less risk of scarring.

69 **A: 3-0 nylon**

The scalp is a tough structure and therefore a medium-strength suture is used; this type of suture also ensures haemostasis as the scalp is very vascular.

70 **F: PDS**

PDS is used for intradermal stitching as it is easy to handle and glides easily.

71 **G: Silk**

Commonly used for drains.

Theme: Testicular disorders

72 **B: Epididymo-orchitis**

Epididymo-orchitis is quite common and torsion very rare after the age of 40 years. These patients require antibiotic cover and a scrotal ultrasound scan to rule out an abscess, which, if persistent, can cause testicular necrosis and will need to be drained.

73 **F: Seminoma**

Seminomas are usually found in 30–40-year-old men. Once suspected, patients should undergo urgent radical orchidectomy as the tumour doubling time is only 28 days. The patient will achieve a complete recovery if treated in time.

74 **G: Testicular torsion**

It is sometimes very difficult to rule out a torsion. However, to be safe rather than sorry, any patient in the 10–20-year-old age group presenting with typical features should undergo exploration, because it only takes 12 hours for the testis to die once it is cut off from its blood supply.

75 **E: Inguinal hernia**

Any scrotal swelling that does not allow you to get above it raises the possibility of an inguinal hernia, and obstruction needs to be excluded.

76 **C: Hydrocele**

In the case of scrotal swellings, if you can get above the swelling it is usually a hydrocele.

Theme: Anorectal disorders

77 **A: Anal fissure**
This usually responds to stool softeners, drinking lots of water and a high-fibre diet. However, a lateral sphincterotomy may need to be performed if these measures fail to remedy the situation.

78 **G: Rectal carcinoma**
Any elderly patient with per rectal bleeding warrants further investigation to rule out cancer. The investigations will involve proctoscopy, rigid and flexible sigmoidoscopy and biopsies.

79 **J: Thrombosed piles**
Can be treated conservatively, but may need operative intervention.

80 **D: Perianal abscess**
This is the classic presentation of a perianal abscess.

81 **B: Fistula-in-ano**
Fistulas are common in patients with Crohn's disease.

Theme: Vomiting in young children

82 **D: Intussusception**
A sausage-shaped mass can sometimes be felt in the abdomen.

83 **E: Meckel's diverticulum**
This is the usual presentation of Meckel's diverticulum.

84 **H: Mid-gut volvulus**
The intestinal distension causes the tenderness with obstruction.

85 **C: Hypertrophic pyloric stenosis**
The biochemical changes that occur are hypochloraemic, hypokalaemic metabolic alkalosis with paradoxical aciduria.

86 **D: Intussusception**
Due to the history of a cold, one should think of enlarged Peyer's patches, which is an underlying cause of intussusception.

Theme: Anatomical landmarks

87 **H: Termination of the spinal cord**
This is the level where the spinal cord ends. Therefore it is an important landmark below which we can perform lumbar punctures or spinal anaesthesia.

88 **I: Transpyloric plane**
The transpyloric plane is an imaginary line perpendicular to the midline that traverses the pylorus and other important structures. It forms one of the boundaries of the abdominal region.

89 **D: Fundus of the gallbladder**
The fundus of the gallbladder is found where the lateral border of the rectus sheath meets with the subcostal margin.

90 **C: Femoral artery pulse is felt**
The mid-inguinal point is the midpoint between the anterior superior iliac spine and the symphysis pubis.

91 **B: Chest-drain insertion**
This is the area for intrathoracic drainage.

Theme: Carcinogens

92 **B: Aniline dyes**
Workers in the rubber and paint industries are exposed to this carcinogen.

93 **G: Nickel**
People working in nickel- and chrome-related industries suffer from this cancer.

94 **C: Asbestos**
Mesothelioma is the coal miners' disease; it is also found in those who work with asbestos.

95 **A: Aflatoxin**
Aflatoxins are produced by *Aspergillus flavus* food moulds.

96 **J: UV light**
UV light is associated with skin cancers.

Theme: Prostate problems

97   **C: Medical management**
In this case the patient could be started on an α-blocker, eg tamsulosin, and reviewed in 6 months' time to see how he responds. Failure to respond would direct him towards TURP (transurethral resection of the prostate).

98   **E: Radical prostatectomy**
The patient seems to be fit and is in the younger age group, with no metastasis. If the patient were older there would be a period of watching and waiting and review of further PSA results.

99   **H: Urodynamics**
This investigation would help us to identify the type of incontinence and plan further management.

100   **B: Hormone therapy**
Patients with advanced cancers are treated with hormones to suppress further tumour growth.

101   **G: TURP**
A failed trial without a catheter means that TURP is the next option.

Theme: Ear problems

102   **G: Wax**
With poor ear hygiene, showering pushes the excess wax nearer to the eardrum.

103   **E: Ototoxicity**
Gentamicin is ototoxic.

104   **B: Acute otitis media**
A purulent discharge from the ear points towards acute otitis media.

105   **A: Acoustic neuroma**
This is associated with *café-au-lait* spots.

106 F: Petrous bone fracture

Head injuries involving the base of the skull can present in this way.

Theme: Jaundiced patients

107 H: Primary sclerosing cholangitis

This is a clinical association and is usually diagnosed by ERCP (endoscopic retrograde cholangiopancreatography) or by transhepatic cholangiography.

108 F: Gilbert's syndrome

Patients with Gilbert's syndrome show a reduced hepatic uptake of bilirubin and reduced activity of bilirubin UDP-glucuronyl transferase. This leads to mild unconjugated hyperbilirubinaemia.

109 A: Acute alcoholic hepatitis

Histological features of alcoholic hepatitis are swollen and necrotic liver cells, infiltration of polymorphs and intracytoplasmic Mallory bodies.

110 F: Liver metastasis

In this case the cancer has metastasised to the liver and may cause biliary obstruction, hence the raised alkaline phosphatase and deranged liver function.

111 C: Charcot's triad (ascending cholangitis)

The three clinical features described together are termed 'Charcot's triad'.

Theme: Dysphagia

112 E: Impacted food bolus

Sudden swallowing of a large food bolus can present in this way.

113 F: Oesophageal carcinoma

A short history of dysphagia and weight loss is highly suggestive of oesophageal malignancy.

114   A: Achalasia
This is a common presentation of achalasia.

115   B: Benign stricture
Long-term reflux disease causes damage to the oesophageal epithelium, which is replaced by fibrosis and results in a stricture. This also predisposes to malignancy.

116   H: Plummer–Vinson syndrome
This is the presentation of Plummer–Vinson syndrome.

Theme: Appropriate use of blood transfusion

117   B: Platelets
Platelets need gentle agitation during storage.

118   B: Platelets
Platelet backup is required during surgery to prevent undue haemorrhage.

119   A: FFP (fresh-frozen plasma)
Such patients need to stop warfarin and need FFP to reverse the action of warfarin.

120   B: Platelets
Collection of platelets is usually done by platelet pooling, whereby it is collected from several donors. (In certain circumstances sensitised patients receive single-donor platelets.)

121   C: RBC
RBC can be stored between 2 °C and 4 °C for up to 4 weeks.

Theme: Acute trauma life support

122   F: Pericardiocentesis
This patient presents with Beck's triad, the signs of cardiac tamponade.

123   D: Intubation
Any patient with a Glasgow Coma Scale (GCS) score below 8 is unable to maintain adequate ventilation and needs support.

124 G: Secondary survey

The patient is stable from the primary survey point of view, and therefore you can continue to perform the secondary survey.

125 C: Guedel airway

A clear airway can be achieved by inserting a Guedel airway.

126 E: Needle thoracocentesis

This is the first-line treatment of a pneumothorax.

Surgery SBAs

1 A 69-year-old man presents with a gradual reduction in urine flow. His PSA is found to be 14.3 µg/l.

What is the most important SINGLE investigation required?

A   Bone scan
B   CT scan
C   Flexible cystoscopy
D   TRUS biopsy
E   USS KUB

2 A 55-year-old heavy smoker presents with pain in his feet at rest. Measurement of his ABPI shows critical ischaemia.

What is the SINGLE best possible management option?

A   Amputation
B   Angiography
C   Conservative plan
D   Duplex scan
E   Heparin

3 A 20-year-old man presents to A&E with sudden-onset pain in his testicles that makes walking difficult.

What is the most urgent SINGLE management option?

A   Antibiotics and analgesia
B   Exploration
C   Orchidopexy
D   Reassurance
E   USS of the testes

4 A 19-year-old woman involved in a motorbike accident presents to resuscitation. Her ABC is stable, but she is found to have an open tibia-fibula fracture on the right side.

What is the most urgent SINGLE management option?

A   Can be left to be operated on the following day
B   Taken to theatre as early as possible
C   Tetanus cover is not required
D   The fractures should be managed conservatively
E   Time of injury bears no importance

5 A 55-year-old woman presents with a thyroid lump and you have a clinical suspicion of follicular carcinoma of the thyroid.

What is the SINGLE best option that fits such a case?

A   Can be managed by lobectomy
B   FNA can differentiate between follicular adenoma and carcinoma
C   Is not seen in this age group
D   Spreads mainly via blood
E   Spreads mainly via lymphatics

6 A 33-year-old woman presents to A&E with an acute abdomen. You are the SHO on call and have come to assess the patient to find out the cause and establish her acute treatment.

What SINGLE sign is not seen in the abdomen?

A   Benedictian sign   D   Shifting dullness
B   Cullen's sign   E   Sister Joseph's nodule
C   Murphy's sign

7 A 35-year-old alcoholic presents to A&E with epigastric pain. At first sight he seems to be jaundiced. You examine him and admit him for further management.

Which SINGLE statement best fits this scenario?

A   ERCP is not used for stenting
B   Gallbladder is never enlarged
C   Raised alkaline phosphatase level denotes liver pathology
D   Unconjugated hyperbilirubinaemia is present in cases of surgical jaundice
E   USS is the first-line investigation

8 A 72-year-old man presented to the clinic with occasional abdominal pain for which his GP could find no reason. After your assessment you organised an USS of the abdomen to rule out any pathology and found that the patient has an abdominal aortic aneurysm.

Which SINGLE statement best applies to AAA?

A   Diameter of less than 5 cm is an indication for surgery
B   Patients present with bilateral flank pain
C   Patients presenting with a leak should be initially assessed by CT scan
D   Repaired by abdominal aortic aneurysmorrhaphy
E   Surveillance is carried out with CT scanning

9 A 17-year-old young woman presents to A&E with severe abdominal pain, mainly around her right loin and iliac fossa, associated with nausea and a single bout of vomiting. She has opened her bowels. She cannot remember her LMP but has recently suffered from cystitis. She used to be a heroin abuser.

Which SINGLE statement best applies here?

A   All such patients should have a nasogastric tube inserted
B   Epigastric pain can mimic MIs
C   Erect chest X-rays always reveal a pneumoperitoneum
D   Patients with loin pain must undergo IVU   USS RUB
E   Young women should not be given a pregnancy test if they present with acute appendicitis

10 A 65-year-old man presents to the clinic with an inguinoscrotal swelling, which he has had for the last 2 years. You have put him down for elective surgery.

Which SINGLE statement best relates to hernias?

A   Direct hernias are less likely to be obstructed
B   Femoral hernias are common in men
C   In women, femoral hernias are commoner than inguinal hernias
D   Littré's hernia means part of the bowel wall is herniating
E   Mesh is used in the shouldice repair

11 A 48-year-old man has sustained a fracture to the mid-arm after falling from a ladder.

Which ONE of the following nerves would be involved?

A Axillary nerve
B Median nerve
C Posterior interosseous nerve
D Radial nerve
E Ulnar nerve

12 A 67-year-old man presents with a painful, swollen right knee that was insidious in onset. You plan to aspirate fluid for analysis.

What is the best position for aspiration of the knee?

A Hip at 45°
B Hip extended
C Knee at 90°
D Knee extended
E Knee in neutral position

13 You are to perform a renal transplant on a patient whose donor is his identical twin brother.

Which is the SINGLE most appropriate term that best describes this type of transplant?

A Alograft   one indiv to another
B Autograft   same indiv
C Isograft   ful twin
D Orthotopic graft   organ t transplanted in @ si   un
E Xenograft   eg. baboon to human

14 A 56-year-old diabetic patient presents with an abscess at the back of his neck with discharging sinuses.

Which ONE of the following terms would you use to describe the presentation?

A Carbuncle
B Cellulitis

C   Faruncle
D   Infected sebaceous cyst
E   Necrotising fasciitis

15 A 45-year-old chronic smoker, who underwent surgery 10 days
ago, has now developed breathlessness.

What is the SINGLE most likely diagnosis?

A   Acute bronchitis
B   Embolism
C   Myocardial infarction
D   Pulmonary oedema
E   Surgical emphysema

16 An 80-year-old woman is admitted with diarrhoea and
vomiting. Stool culture shows her to be positive for *Clostridium
difficile* toxin.

Which is the SINGLE most appropriate description of this organism?

A   Gram-negative cocci
B   Gram-negative rods
C   Gram-positive cocci
D   Gram-positive rods
E   Spirochaete

17 A 45-year-old welder presents with a metal splinter in his eye.

*What is the SINGLE best management option you can offer in the
A&E setting?*

A   Eye wash
B   Immediate ophthalmology referral
C   Removal of the foreign body under magnification
D   Retinoscopy
E   Topical antibiotic

Surgery SBAs – Answers

1 D: TRUS biopsy
A raised PSA is an indicator of concern, and prostate cancer needs to be ruled out at the earliest opportunity by taking biopsies for histopathology.

2 B: Angiography
Once a limb has been diagnosed as critical, the decision on how best to manage the case needs to be made. Angiography will delineate the extent of stenosis and tell us if there is a good enough inflow and run-off to proceed to bypass surgery.

3 B: Exploration
Young men with such a presentation should be taken for exploration immediately, as time means death of the testis. You have nothing to lose if it is a false alarm.

4 B: Taken to theatre as early as possible
Here again, lost time means an increase in the risk of grave infection. Such a case must take top priority, even if this means negotiating with general surgeons who are also in the queue for performing an operation.

5 D: Spreads mainly via blood
The opposites of all the other options are correct.

6 A: Benedictian sign
This is a sign of median nerve palsy.

7 E: USS is the first-line investigation
Ultrasound scanning is quick, non-invasive and provides much information with regard to the hepatobiliary system. A raised alkaline phosphatase level denotes bile duct pathology, and ERCP is used for stenting. Surgical jaundice presents with a rise in the conjugated type of bilirubin. The gallbladder can be enlarged according to Courvoisier's law.

8   E: Surveillance is carried out with CT scanning

A diameter of more than 5 cm is an indication for surgery. Monitoring is done with the help of USS. Patients present with central and upper abdominal pain radiating to their backs, and patients with leaking aneurysms should be taken to theatre immediately.

9   B: Epigastric pain can mimic MIs

All women of reproductive age should be given a pregnancy test to rule out an ectopic pregnancy. NG tubes are indicated for patients who are vomiting, especially in cases of bowel obstruction where aspiration of the contents and bowel rest is required. Patients with loin pain and high creatinine levels should undergo ultrasound scanning of the kidneys, ureters and bladder (USS KUB) and not intravenous urography (IVU). This is because the kidneys are not in a fit state to excrete the dye effectively, therefore giving inaccurate results. Always remember that heroin addicts are known to suffer myocardial infarcts (MIs) at a younger age than usual.

10   D: Littré's hernia means that part of the bowel wall is herniating

Littré's hernia means the content is Meckel's diverticulum.

11   D: Radial nerve

The patient has sustained a mid-shaft humeral fracture and this would involve the radial nerve, which spirals around the back of the humeral shaft.

12   D: Knee extended

When aspirating a knee joint the knee should be extended and the needle inserted laterally and below the patella.

13   C: Isograft

Grafts performed between identical twins are termed 'isografts'.

14   A: Carbuncle

Carbuncles are subcutaneous collections of pus that discharge to the surface via multiple sinuses. They are is usually caused by staphylococcal infection.

15 B: Embolism

The history is quite typical of embolism, which is most common after major surgery and should be prevented pre-, intra-, and postoperatively with the help of TED stockings, pneumatic calf compression and low molecular weight heparin.

16 D: Gram-positive rods

Clostridium difficile are Gram-positive rods with a characteristic drumstick appearance due to the presence of spores.

17 C: Removal of the foreign body under magnification

Foreign bodies in the eye are usually easy to remove under magnification. Topical antibiotics are given and the eye is covered with an eye pad. The patient is later reviewed by the ophthalmologists as an outpatient.

Obstetrics and Gynaecology

Chapter contributed by
Jayanta Chatterjee MBBS DFFP DRCOG

Obstetrics and Gynaecology EMQs

Theme: **Bleeding in pregnancy**

Options

A	Abruption of placenta secondary to pre-eclampsia	F	Placenta accreta
B	Antepartum haemorrhage	G	Placenta praevia
C	Concealed haemorrhage	H	Preterm labour
D	In labour	I	Primary postpartum haemorrhage
E	Intrauterine death	J	Secondary postpartum haemorrhage

Instructions

For each of the patients described below choose the SINGLE most appropriate diagnosis from the list of options above. Each option may be used once, more than once or not at all.

1 A 25-year-old woman, who is 38 weeks' pregnant, presents to the labour ward with a history of fewer fetal movements than usual during the evening. She also says that abdominal contractions are coming every few minutes and she has been having a bloodstained show per vagina for the last few minutes. On vaginal examination: cervix is fully effaced, 9-cm dilated, cephalic presentation and station is +1. ☐

2 A 30-year-old primigravida, who is 30 weeks' pregnant, presents to the labour ward with absent fetal movements. She also complains of severe headache, heartburn and seeing floaters before her eyes for the last few days. On examination: BP, 170/110 mmHg; urine, protein ++++; rock-hard uterus with no visible signs of fetal movements per abdomen. ☐

3 A 20-year-old pregnant woman, 32/40 weeks by date, presents to the antenatal clinic with a history of painless per vaginal bleeding after intercourse. On examination: P/A – soft and relaxed, uterus = dates; cardiotocograph (CTG) – reactive.

4 A 24-year-old primigravida, who is 30 weeks' pregnant, presents to the labour ward with a history of constant abdominal pain for the last few hours. She also gives a history of having lost a cupful of fresh blood per vagina before the pain started. Abdominal examination shows an irritable uterus. CTG – reactive.

5 A 38-year-old woman, 10 days' postpartum, presents to her GP with a history of a foul-smelling discharge per vagina. She also gives a history of passing blood clots per vagina since yesterday. On examination her BP is 90/40 mmHg, pulse 110 bpm, temperature 38 °C; P/A, uterus tender on palpation and fundus 2 cm above the umbilicus; P/S, blood clots +++.

Theme: **Bleeding per vagina**

Options

A	Acute appendicitis
B	Atrophic vaginitis
C	Cervical cancer
D	Cervical polyp
E	Complete miscarriage
F	Ectopic pregnancy
G	Endometrial cancer
H	Endometrial polyp
I	Incomplete miscarriage
J	Threatened miscarriage
K	Toxic-shock syndrome

Instructions

For each of the patients described below choose the SINGLE most appropriate diagnosis from the list of options above. Each option may be used once, more than once or not at all.

6 A 56-year-old, postmenopausal woman comes to your GP surgery with a 2-week history of sudden-onset bleeding per vagina. She describes the bleeding to be very, very heavy and having to use 7–10 sanitary towels every day. She has suffered from breast cancer in the past and was treated with surgery, radiotherapy and chemotherapy. She was also on tamoxifen for 5 years and was given the 'all clear' only last year. ☐

7 A 23-year-old woman presents to A&E with a history of postcoital bleeding. She describes the bleeding to be more of a spotting. ☐

8 A 72-year-old woman comes to the gynaecological clinic with a history of vaginal bleeding. She complains of having had spotting for a couple of days but this has now completely resolved. On examination the vulva looks red and inflamed. ☐

9 A 17-year-old girl presents to A&E with a sudden-onset right iliac fossa pain radiating to the umbilicus. She first noticed the pain last night and it has got progressively worse. She lives with her present boyfriend and also gives a history of her period being overdue for a couple of days. On examination her temperature is 37.5 °C, pulse 90 bpm, BP 110/68 mmHg. Per abdominal examination shows guarding and tenderness at the right iliac fossa. Pregnancy test (PAT) is negative; urinalysis shows leucocytes +. ☐

10 A 28-year-old woman presents to A&E in a state of shock. She is in severe pain and gives a history of spotting per vagina and feeling unwell for the last few days. Today, the bleeding has become very heavy and she has had to use several tampons. She has also passed some 'livery' bits, forcing her to come to the hospital. She is known to suffer from irregular periods and her partner has had a vasectomy. On examination her pulse is 120 bpm, BP 100/70 mmHg, temperature 40 °C and GCS score is 7. ☐

Theme: **Gynaecological investigations**

Options

A   Cervical punch biopsy
B   Colposcopy and LLETZ
C   Diagnostic hysteroscopy and
    endometrial biopsy
D   Diagnostic laparoscopy and
    tubal dye test
E   Diagnostic laparotomy
F   Hycosy   *day 8 – 10*
G   Hysterosalpingography

H   Pregnancy test and serum
    βHCG
I   Serum LH and serum FSH
J   Transabdominal USS of the
    pelvis
K   Transvaginal USS of the pelvis,
    Pippele® biopsy and saline
    sonography

Instructions

For each of the patients described below choose the SINGLE most
appropriate investigation from the list of options above. Each option may
be used once, more than once or not at all.

11 A 55-year-old woman comes to your gynaecological clinic with
a history of intermenstrual bleeding while on cyclical combined
HRT. □

12 A 23-year-old woman is rushed into A&E in a state of shock.
Her partner informs you that she had been complaining of
lower abdominal pain this morning and then suddenly
collapsed. He also tells you that her LMP was 6–7 weeks ago. A
portable TAS shows free fluid in the pelvis. On examination her
GCS score is 3, pulse 140 bpm, BP 70/40 mmHg. □

13 A 35-year-old patient comes to your clinic with a 2-year history
of primary subfertility. She also gives a history of menstrual
irregularity, severe dysmenorrhoea and dyspareunia. □

14 A 42-year-old woman comes to your clinic with a 4-year history of secondary infertility. She already has a 6-year-old girl who was conceived after IVF treatment. It has only been recently that she has had the financial means to seriously consider a second child. She also informs you that for the last few months her periods have gradually become more and more irregular and she has also been experiencing night sweats. ☐

15 A 48-year-old asylum seeker presents to your clinic with a history of a bloodstained, foul-smelling vaginal discharge. On per speculum examination you see a large ulcerated mass arising from the cervix. ☐

Theme: **Pelvic pain**

Options

A   Acute PID
B   Appendicitis
C   Chronic PID
D   Diverticulitis
E   Ectopic pregnancy
F   Endometriosis

G   Pyelonephritis
H   Red degeneration of fibroid
I   Torsion of ovarian cyst
J   Ureteric calculi
K   Urinary tract infection

Instructions

For each of the patients described below choose the SINGLE most appropriate diagnosis from the list of options above. Each option may be used once, more than once or not at all.

16 A 23-year-old woman, who is 6 months' pregnant, presents to the labour ward with a 2-day history of right lower abdominal pain and diarrhoea. On examination the uterus is soft and she is very tender over the right loin. Her temperature is 38.9 °C and pulse 110 bpm. Urine shows protein ++, leucocytes +, and no nitrates. ☐

17 A 55-year-old woman presents to A&E complaining of severe left iliac fossa pain. She is also noted to have a low-grade temperature with guarding and tenderness in the left side of her abdomen. While taking a history you gather that, although she is now menopausal, she has suffered from heavy periods, due to her fibroids, in the past. She gives no urinary symptoms but has been constipated recently. ☐

18 A 35-year-old multigravida, who is 7 months' pregnant, presents to the labour ward complaining of severe abdominal pain. She is requiring morphine injections for pain control. On examination her uterus is 36 weeks' gestation and soft. CTG is reactive, with plenty of fetal movements. ☐

19 An 18-year-old woman comes to A&E complaining of severe lower abdominal pain. She is on the combined pill but has been noticing breakthrough bleeding in-between her cycles. On examination she is febrile with generalised lower abdominal tenderness. Vaginal examination shows that cervical excitation is positive, with purulent vaginal discharge. ☐

20 A 26-year-old woman comes to the gynaecological emergency clinic with a 1-year history of pelvic pain. She informs you that she has been investigated in the past for pelvic pain by diagnostic laparoscopy, when they noticed that she had a right ovarian chocolate cyst. ☐

Theme: **Contraception**

Options

A	Combined oral contraceptive pills	G	Intrauterine copper device
B	Condoms	H	Lactational amenorrhoea method (LAM)
C	Dianette®	I	Levonorgestrel ('morning-after pill')
D	Diaphragm with spermicidal gel	J	Mirena® coil
E	Implanon®	K	Progesterone-only pill
F	Injection of Depo-Provera®		

Instructions

For each of the patients described below choose the SINGLE most appropriate method of contraception from the list of options above. Each option may be used once, more than once or not at all.

21 A 16-year-old girl comes to your family planning clinic requesting contraceptive advice. She has been sexually active for the past year and is in a stable relationship with her boyfriend. She also informs you that she does not want anything that will make her acne worse.

22 A 26-year-old woman, 7 weeks' postpartum, comes to your family planning clinic for contraceptive advice. While taking a history from her you gather that she is partially breast-feeding, although the vast majority of the feeds are breast-feeds. She is not keen on any hormonal contraceptive, as her friends have told her that they can reduce breast milk.

23 A 24-year-old woman tourist is brought into A&E by the police surgeon who informs you that she was raped 4 days ago. You are asked to perform a medical examination on the patient and advise her about the most suitable contraception.

24 A 45-year-old woman comes to your clinic requesting sterilisation. While taking a history, you gather that she has been happily married for the last 20 years and her husband is not keen on a vasectomy. She also tells you that she has recently noticed that her periods have become heavier and puts this down to her increased weight. Her present BMI is 38.

25 A 35-year-old woman comes to your family planning clinic requesting contraceptive advice. She has five children and does not want any more. Her last two pregnancies were conceived after contraception failure, while on the pill and the injection. Looking through her past records you notice that she had been tested positive for *Chlamydia* and was seen in the GUM clinic 2 years ago.

Theme: **Infertility/assisted reproductive technology**

Options

A	Donor insemination	G	Laparoscopic multi-electrocauterisation of the ovary
B	GIFT/ZIFT (gamete/zygote intrafallopian transfer)	H	Ovulation induction with follicular tracking
C	IUI (intrauterine insemination)		
D	IVF	I	Surrogacy
E	IVF with donor egg	J	Tubal surgery
F	IVF with ICSI (*in vitro* fertilisation with intracytoplasmic sperm injection)		

Instructions

For each of the infertile couples described below choose the most appropriate management from the list given above. Each option may be used once, more than once or not at all.

26 A 38-year-old woman and a 40-year-old man come to your infertility clinic for advice. They have been married for the last 6 years and have been trying for a baby for the last 3 years. Initial investigations show a normal Hycosy and endocrine profile for the woman, while the man's semen analysis shows him to have oligoasthenospermia. ☐

27 A 23-year-old woman and a 28-year-old man come to your infertility clinic giving a 1-year history of primary infertility. While taking a history from the man you gather he was diagnosed as a child to have hypospadias. ☐

28 A 28-year-old woman and a 30-year-old man come to your fertility clinic giving an 18-month history of primary infertility. Initial endocrine tests show the woman has anovulatory cycles while her partner's semen analysis is normal. ☐

29 A 30-year-old woman and a 35-year-old man come to your fertility clinic for advice. Unfortunately, the woman has lost both fallopian tubes due to recurrent ectopic pregnancies. □

30 A 30-year-old woman and her 42-year-old partner come to your infertility clinic for advice. The woman informs you that they have a 4-year-old son, and during his birth she had a massive haemorrhage due to placenta praevia and ended up with a Caesarean hysterectomy. They now want a second child. □

Theme: **Sexually transmitted infections (STIs)**

Options

A	Chancroid	G	Herpes simplex
B	Condyloma acuminata	H	Herpes zoster
C	Gonorrhoea	I	HIV
D	Granuloma inguinale	J	Lymphogranuloma venereum
E	Hepatitis B		(LGV)
F	Hepatitis C	K	Syphilitic primary chancre

(handwritten annotations: H. ducreyi – painful; HPV, warts; Donovan bodies; infect mononucleosis; painless; Frei's test)

Instructions

For each of the patients described below choose the SINGLE most appropriate diagnosis from the list of options above. Each option may be used once, more than once or not at all.

31 A 29-year-old asylum seeker from Sub-Saharan Africa comes to the GUM clinic with a history of a painful ulcer on the prepuce of his penis that he has noticed for the last few days. On examination you notice a deep, large ulcer with well-defined margins on the prepuce. You also notice a few smaller satellite ulcers on the glans penis with tender swollen inguinal lymph nodes. ☐

32 A 22-year-old truck driver comes to the GUM clinic complaining of a flu-like illness with fever, headache and backache. He has also noticed a few small, fluid-filled, itchy blisters on his genital area. He also complains of severe burning during micturition. ☐

33 A 36-year-old homosexual patient comes to the GUM clinic requesting treatment for the white plaques in his mouth. While examining the patient you notice a few bluish-brown nodules on his arm. ☐

34 A 22-year-old woman comes to A&E feeling unwell and with a high fever. While taking a history you gather she has a vaginal discharge, dysuria and painful intercourse. While examining the patient you notice a large lump in the vulval area, which her GP has diagnosed to be a Bartholin's abscess. ☐

35 A 38-year-old intravenous drug user is brought to A&E in a comatose state. On examination you identify signs suggestive of chronic liver disease with jaundice and ascites. When the results of the tests for viral markers are back later, you notice he is positive for HBsAg and anti-HBe.

Theme: **Vaginal discharge**

Options

A	Atrophic vaginitis	G	Gonorrhoea
B	Bacterial vaginosis (BV)	H	Mittelschmerz
C	Candidiasis	I	Non-gonococcal urethritis (NGU)
D	Cervical cancer	J	*Trichomonas vaginalis* (TV)
E	Ectropion	K	Vulvovaginitis
F	Foreign body		

Instructions

For each of the patients described below choose the SINGLE most appropriate diagnosis from the list of options above. Each option may be used once, more than once or not at all.

36 A 5-year-old girl is brought by her mother to the walk-in clinic. The mother informs you that she has been recently noticing a discharge on the girl's undergarments. On examination of the external genitalia you notice it to be red and inflamed. ☐

37 A 65-year-old woman comes to your gynaecology outpatient clinic to have her ring pessary changed. While taking a history from her you gather that, although she has been fine with regards to her prolapse, she has recently been having some bloodstained discharge. ☐

38 A 23-year-old woman comes to your GP surgery complaining of an itchy vaginal discharge. She is in a stable relationship and is not on any contraceptive pills. On examination you notice red and oedematous labia with white spongy areas. ☐

39 An 18-year-old woman comes to your GP surgery complaining of excessive vaginal discharge. She is on the combined pill and describes her symptoms as 'feeling wet all the time'. ☐

40 A 26-year-old woman comes to the clinic complaining of dysuria and painful intercourse. While taking a history from her, she tells you she has been recently getting a funny vaginal discharge. She describes it as being frothy with a musty smell, causing intense itching and soreness in her vagina.

Theme: **Endocrine disorders**

Options

A	Congenital adrenal hyperplasia (CAH)	F	Multiple endocrine neoplasia (MEN)
B	Craniopharyngioma	G	Nelson's syndrome
C	Graves' disease	H	Polycystic ovarian syndrome (PCOS)
D	Hashimoto's thyroiditis		
E	Hypogonadotrophic hypogonadism (Kallmann's syndrome)	I	Premature gonadal failure
		J	Prolactinoma
		K	Sheehan's syndrome

Instructions

For each of the patients described below choose the SINGLE most appropriate diagnosis from the list of options above. Each option may be used once, more than once or not at all.

41 A mother brings her 6-month-old child to the paediatric A&E complaining of vomiting and weight loss. On examination the child appears emaciated and lethargic. You also notice the child has clitoral hypertrophy and labioscrotal fusion. Initial blood tests show her U&E to be deranged, with a low sodium and high potassium level. $\downarrow Na \quad \uparrow k$

42 A 22-year-old man is referred to your endocrine clinic by his GP with the complaint of feeling a lump in the front of his neck that he suspects to be a thyroid goitre. While taking a history you gather that he recently dropped out of university because he was unable to cope with the curriculum. He also complains of eye discomfort when he is watching the television. On examination you notice him to be rather tall, with a BMI of 18.

43 An 18-year-old man comes to the ophthalmology clinic complaining of headache and visual disturbances. He has been getting worsening headaches for the past few months. On general physical examination you note him to very short and obese with no secondary sexual features. Visual field examination shows him to have a bitemporal hemianopia.

44 A 23-year-old Asian man comes to the infertility clinic complaining of difficulty in having intercourse. On questioning, you gather that he fails to get a proper erection. You also learn there are other members of his family with similar problems. ☐

45 A 26-year-old woman comes to the outpatient clinic complaining of amenorrhoea for the last 2 months. A pregnancy test is negative. She tells you that her periods had become very light and irregular before they stopped. Her skin has also been getting greasy and spotty. Endocrine tests show her to have raised serum LH and prolactin levels, a normal serum FSH level and low levels of SHBG. ☐

Theme: **Chromosomal abnormalities**

Options

A	Christmas disease	G	Klinefelter's syndrome
B	Cystic fibrosis	H	Myotonic dystrophy
C	Fragile X syndrome	I	Patau's syndrome Tri 13
D	Haemochromatosis	J	Sickle cell disease AR
E	Hereditary spherocytosis AD	K	Turner's syndrome
F	Huntington's disease AD		

Instructions

For each of the disorders described below choose the SINGLE most appropriate diagnosis from the list of options above. Each option may be used once, more than once or not at all.

46 Low-set ears, cleft lip and palate, polydactyly, micro-ophthalmia and mental retardation. Babies rarely survive for more than a few weeks. ☐

47 Autosomal dominant, triple-repeat expansion disorder affecting chromosome 4. ☐

48 Autosomal recessive, single-gene disorder on chromosome 11, causing childhood anaemia and jaundice. ☐

49 Decreased crown-pubis:pubis-heel ratio. Associated with decreased libido, infertility and gynaecomastia and mental retardation, but affected individuals have a normal lifespan. ☐

50 Sex-linked chromosomal disorder. It is the most common inherited cause of mental retardation in men. Associated with macro-orchidism. ☐

Theme: **Vulval disorders**

Options

A	Behçet's disease	G	Sebaceous cyst
B	Carcinoma of the vulva	H	Varicose veins
C	Condyloma lata	I	Vulval abscess
D	Herpes simplex	J	Vulval psoriasis
E	Leucoplakia	K	Vulval wart
F	Lichen sclerosis		

Instructions

For each of the patients described below choose the SINGLE most appropriate diagnosis from the list of options above. Each option may be used once, more than once or not at all.

51 A 55-year-old woman comes to the outpatient department complaining of vaginal bleeding. She also tells you that she has recently noticed a small ulcer on her genitals. On examination you notice an ulcer on the vulva, which has an indurated base and everted margins. You can also palpate inguinal lymphadenopathy.

52 A 30-year-old, 7-months' pregnant woman comes to the antenatal clinic complaining of a bluish lump that she has noticed in her vulva. The lump has gradually increased in size but has remained painless.

53 A 28-year-old woman comes to the gynaecology clinic having noticed white patches, which are itchy, on her vulva. On examination you notice the vulval skin to be thickened in the areas with the white patches.

54 A 20-year-old patient, who is 6 months' pregnant, attends the GUM clinic having been referred by the community midwife after noticing warty lesions on her vulva. On taking a history you gather she is in a stable relationship and has noticed this growth only in the last few weeks. She has no history of having a sexually transmitted infection in the past.

55 A 32-year-old woman is referred by her GP with a painful vulval swelling, which has become progressively larger and has now burst. On examining her you notice a lump in the labia majora. The lump has a punctum and is discharging foul-smelling pus. ☐

Theme: **Gynaecological surgery**

Options

A	Burch colposuspension	G	McDonald's suture
B	Fenton's procedure	H	Shirodkar's suture
C	Kelly's plication	I	Tension-free vaginal tape (TVT)
D	LeFort operation	J	Wertheim's surgery
E	Manchester's operation	K	Zacharin procedure
F	Marsupialisation		

Instructions

For each of the descriptions mentioned below match the SINGLE most likely operation from the list of options above. Each option may be used once, more than once or not at all.

56 Amputation of the cervix with anterior colporrhaphy and posterior colpoperineorrhaphy.

57 Everting the inner cyst wall by suturing it to the vaginal mucosa with interrupted sutures.

58 Application of a reinforcing band around the cervix, beneath the mucosa, at the level of the internal os after reflection of the bladder.

59 Repair of a vaginal vault prolapse after hysterectomy.

60 Removal of the uterus, tubes and ovaries, along with the top of the vagina, and includes pelvic and para-aortic lymph node clearance.

Theme: **Abdominal swellings**

Options

A	Adenomyosis	G	Ovarian malignancy
B	Aortic aneurysm	H	Ovarian teratoma
C	Fibroid uterus	I	Spigelian hernia
D	Haematometra	J	Strangulated hernia
E	Krukenburg tumour	K	Tubo-ovarian abscess
F	Ovarian hyperstimulation syndrome (OHSS)		

Instructions

For each of the patients described below choose the SINGLE most appropriate diagnosis from the list of options above. Each option may be used once, more than once or not at all.

61 A 26-year-old woman is referred to A&E by her GP with a history of breathlessness and abdominal swelling. On taking a history you gather that she has been having fertility treatment. ☐

62 While operating on a 28-year-old woman for torsion of an ovarian cyst, you notice fatty material with a few tufts of hair coming out from the cyst. ☐

63 A 35-year-old Afro-Caribbean woman comes to the gynaecology clinic complaining of severe dysmenorrhoea. On vaginal bimanual examination you find a bulky uterus with no other significant findings. While looking through her notes you gather that she recently had a diagnostic laparoscopy for pelvic pain where the findings were all normal. ☐

64 A 42-year-old woman presents to A&E with an acute abdomen. While examining her you notice she is obese with a lax abdominal wall due to her multiparity. On abdominal palpation you notice a firm and tender lump lateral to the umbilicus that cannot be reduced. There is abdominal guarding and rigidity with absent bowel sounds. Vital signs: pulse 100 bpm, BP 100/70 mmHg and temperature 38 °C. ☐

65 A 15-year-old girl comes to A&E with abdominal pain. On abdominal examination you notice a tender, palpable mass. While taking a menstrual history you gather that she has not started menstruating yet.

Theme: **Obstetric emergencies**

Options

A	Amniotic fluid embolism	F	Placental abruption
B	Atonic postpartum haemorrhage (PPH)	G	Pulmonary embolism
		H	Shoulder dystocia
C	Cord prolapse	I	Uterine hyperstimulation
D	Fetal distress	J	Uterine inversion
E	Perineal trauma	K	Uterine rupture

Instructions

For each of the clinical scenarios described below choose the SINGLE most appropriate diagnosis from the list of options above. Each option may be used once, more than once or not at all.

66 While you are on-call on the labour ward you are asked to help at a delivery in one of the rooms. On entering the room you notice the woman delivering with 'turtling' of the baby's head. ☐

67 While on-call on the labour ward you are urgently summoned to one of the delivery rooms. The attending midwife quickly briefs you that the patient has just delivered a 5-kg baby and after placental delivery has continued to bleed profusely. On examination you find the uterus to be hard and contracted. ☐

68 While on-call on the labour ward you are crash-bleeped to see one of the labouring patients. On entering the room you note fetal bradycardia on the CTG. While quickly reviewing the patient's notes, you gather this is her second pregnancy and her last delivery was by Caesarean section 2 years ago. ☐

69 While on-call for obstetrics you are crash-bleeped to see a patient who has suddenly collapsed in the postnatal ward. The midwife informs you that the patient had a Caesarean section 5 days ago and was due to be discharged tomorrow. ☐

70 While on-call on the labour ward you are urgently asked to review a patient who has just delivered. On entering the room you find the patient to be in a state of shock. The attending midwife informs you that the patient suddenly collapsed after delivery of the placenta. On abdominal palpation you find it hard to outline the uterine fundus.

Theme: **Breast disorders**

Options

A	Acute mastitis	G	Fibroadenoma
B	Benign breast cyst	H	Fibroadenosis
C	Breast abscess	I	Galactocele
D	Breast cancer	J	Lipoma
E	Duct ectasia	K	Sebaceous cyst
F	Fat necrosis		

Instructions

For each of the patients described below choose the SINGLE most appropriate diagnosis from the list of options above. Each option may be used once, more than once or not at all.

71 A 28-year-old woman comes to the GP surgery complaining of a lump in her breast. On examination you notice a non-tender, firm, mobile mass in the right upper quadrant of her breast. ☐

72 A 65-year-old woman comes to the GP surgery complaining that she recently noticed a change in the shape of her left breast. On examination you notice skin dimpling and a *peau-d'orange* appearance of her skin over the left lower quadrant. ☐

73 A 55-year-old woman comes to her GP surgery complaining that she has recently noticed a change in the shape of her nipple. On examination you note her nipple to be slit-like with no discharge or change in colour. ☐

74 A 26-year-old woman comes to A&E complaining of pain in her right breast. On examination you notice severe tenderness and swelling in the periareolar area. You also find her axillary lymph nodes to be swollen. Her vital signs are stable, although she is running a high temperature. ☐

75 A 33-year-old woman comes to see her GP, worried about lumps in her breast. She is very anxious and informs her GP that recently she has noticed two lumps in her breast. On examination you notice a few smooth, ill-defined, soft lumps in the outer quadrant of her breast.

Theme: **High-risk pregnancy**

Options

A   Cervical suture
B   Immediate delivery
C   Intravenous antibiotics
D   Intravenous ritodrine
E   Low-dose aspirin
F   Low-dose heparin
G   Prophylactic oral antibiotics

H   Screening for bacterial vaginosis
I   Serial cervical-length assessment
    by transvaginal scan
J   Serial growth scans
K   Twice-weekly umbilical artery
    Doppler and AFI measurement

Instructions

For each of the patients described below choose the SINGLE most appropriate management from the list of options above. Each option may be used once, more than once or not at all.

76 A pregnant woman of 34 weeks comes to the labour ward with abdominal pain and contractions which she has been experiencing for the last few hours. While looking through her notes you gather she is a carrier for group-B *Streptococcus* (GBS). Vaginal examination reveals she is 4-cm dilated. ☐

77 A 35-weeks pregnant woman is referred from the fetal medicine unit to the antenatal clinic. A routine growth scan has shown that fetal growth has fallen from the 10th centile to below the 3rd centile on the customised growth chart. The scan also shows the AFI to be greatly reduced, although the umbilical artery Doppler is normal. ☐

78 A 12-weeks pregnant woman comes to the antenatal clinic for her booking visit. This is her second pregnancy and, unfortunately, she lost her last pregnancy at 22 weeks' gestation. While reviewing her notes you gather that she came in on that occasion with a history of abdominal pain for a few hours and soon afterwards she ruptured her membranes and delivered. ☐

79 An 8-weeks pregnant woman comes to the antenatal clinic for her booking visit. She is very anxious, as this is her fourth pregnancy and she has had three spontaneous miscarriages before. She has been investigated in the recurrent miscarriage clinic and tests showed she had very low levels of IgG anticardiolipin antibodies (aCL).   ☐

80 A 20-weeks pregnant woman comes to the antenatal clinic for her booking visit. She is a G3P2, having had her previous two deliveries preterm at 34 and 35 weeks.   ☐

Theme: **Prescribing in pregnancy**

Options

A	Atenolol	G	Methyldopa
B	Cefalexin	H	Misoprostol per rectum
C	Cisplatin	I	Oral mifepristone
D	Diazepam	J	Tetracycline
E	Magnesium sulphate	K	Trimethoprim
F	Methotrexate		

Instructions

For each of the clinical scenarios described below choose the SINGLE most appropriate treatment from the list of options given above. Each option can be used once, more than once or not at all.

81 A 28-year-old 26-weeks pregnant woman presents to the labour ward with off-and-on abdominal pain and burning on micturition. On examination, you feel regular uterine contractions and she has suprapubic tenderness. Dipstick urinalysis shows leucocytes +++, +ve for nitrate, and blood and protein ++.

82 A 30-year-old 8-weeks pregnant woman comes to the antenatal clinic for her booking visit. She is known to have essential hypertension and was previously on an ACE inhibitor, which she has stopped ever since she found out that she was pregnant. The GP has referred her to you to advise about alternative medication.

83 While on-call on the labour ward you are asked to attend to a patient who is having a massive postpartum haemorrhage (PPH) after a normal delivery. The first- and second-line drugs have been used without much success.

84 A 26-year-old woman comes to the early pregnancy unit with a 6-week history of amenorrhoea and a positive pregnancy test. A diagnosis is made on transvaginal scan of right tubal ectopic pregnancy. After doing her βHCG levels, she is found to be suitable for medical management.

85 A 30-weeks pregnant lady presents to the labour ward with constant headache, epigastric pain and seeing halos. She is also noticed to be very jittery and examination of her reflexes elicits clonus. Her BP is 136/90mmHg and urine examination shows protein ++++.

Obstetrics and Gynaecology EMQs – Answers

Theme: Bleeding in pregnancy

1 **D: In labour**
This is clearly a question to test one's practical obstetric knowledge. The first sentence is slightly confusing for people with no obstetric experience. It is important to analyse the information given in this clinical scenario. Any pregnancy that progresses beyond 37 weeks is considered to be term. Normally, the fetal movements are felt less as the presenting part of the fetus becomes engaged in the pelvis as the labour progresses. The cervical findings are typically found during the first stage of established labour (basic obstetrics). The bloodstained show is found when the presenting part of the fetus (the head) compresses on the cervix to make it effaced (thinned) and dilated. This is, once again, a normal finding in the late first stage of labour.

2 **A: Abruption of the placenta secondary to pre-eclampsia**
Once again it is important to analyse the information provided. There are two important aspects to consider in this scenario. The history of headache, heartburn and visual symptoms, together with the findings of raised blood pressure and urinary protein are diagnostic of pre-eclampsia. The clinical feature of a rock-hard uterus is secondary to placental abruption, which is due to pre-eclampsia. Although the mention of no visible fetal movements may make one think about option E (intrauterine death), it is important not to make presumptions and answer only on the basis of the information provided. The diagnosis of intrauterine death is made only in the absence of a fetal heartbeat on ultrasound scanning.

3 **G: Placenta praevia**
This is a classic presentation of placenta praevia. 'Antepartum

haemorrhage' is the broad term for bleeding during the antenatal period. However, painless, postcoital bleeding is pathological of placenta praevia.

4   B: Antepartum haemorrhage
The clinical features that require emphasis here are the constant abdominal pain, bleeding per vagina and irritable uterus. This is probably due to a small abruption. The difference in this question from the previous one is the mention of painful bleeding per vagina, in contrast to the previous scenario of painless vaginal bleeding.

5   J: Secondary postpartum haemorrhage
The difference between primary and secondary postpartum haemorrhage is the timing of bleeding after delivery. Primary PPH usually occurs 24–48 hours after delivery, while secondary PPH can occur from 48 hours up to 14 days after delivery. In this clinical scenario, secondary PPH is due to endometritis (an infection caused by bacterial penetration of the residual stratum basalis of the endometrium), as the raised temperature, offensive vaginal discharge and tender uterus suggests. The underlying aggravating factor may be due to retained products of conception, which provides a rich culture medium for the growth of bacteria.

Theme: Bleeding per vagina

6   G: Endometrial cancer
Approximately 10% of women presenting to the clinic with postmenopausal bleeding prove to have endometrial cancer. The clinical picture of a sudden presentation with heavy bleeding and a history of tamoxifen use are important clues leading to the diagnosis. Tamoxifen is an oestrogen-receptor antagonist, which is the adjuvant hormonal therapy of choice in women with oestrogen receptor-positive breast cancer. One important side-effect of oestrogens is endometrial changes, and hence they are generally used in combination with progestogens.

7   D: Cervical polyp
This is fairly straightforward. The other differential diagnosis for postcoital bleeding is cancer of the cervix, which is easily excluded

considering the age of the patient and her presentation. Young women using the combined pill are more prone to polyps and cervical erosions, due to the action of oestrogen on the squamous epithelium.

8   B: Atrophic vaginitis
Once again the signs of a red, inflamed and thin vulva are tell-tale signs of the diagnosis. The treatment is a local oestrogen cream.

9   A: Acute appendicitis
The fact that the urine pregnancy test is negative makes the diagnosis very simple. *You cannot be pregnant if your pregnancy test is negative. Hence, you cannot have an ectopic pregnancy.*

10   K: Toxic-shock syndrome
This is a slightly tricky question as a lot of information is thrown at you and it is important to decipher which points are relevant to the question. Remember, there are no trick questions in this examination. Although you can be misled to think that this question may be related to miscarriage, the last sentence in the scenario rules out that possibility fairly convincingly. The term 'livery bits' is a typical term used by patients to describe blood clots. The clinical findings of a very high temperature and a markedly raised pulse rate take you towards the diagnosis of some sort of infection as the underlying cause. The mention of tampons clinches your diagnosis. Toxic-shock syndrome is caused by vaginal colonisation by toxigenic staphylococci. This was first noticed in the 1980s in healthy, young menstruating women who used tampons. The absorbent tampons create conditions favourable to the multiplication of organisms and toxin production. This multisystem, and occasionally near-fatal, condition can occur in any non-immune individual infected by the TSST-1-producing strain.

Theme: **Gynaecological investigations**

11   K: Transvaginal USS of the pelvis, Pippele® biopsy and saline sonography
Although you might think that any of options C, J, or K may be

right, in the NHS setting this is the most appropriate answer. Most hospitals have these one-stop 'Postmenopausal bleeding clinics' where the diagnostic procedures are performed on an outpatient basis. Sonohysterography is gradually replacing outpatient hysteroscopy as it can be combined with the scan to give a more detailed pelvic assessment. It is also more patient-friendly. The most likely diagnosis in this case is endometrial polyp, which is common combined HRT users.

12   E: Diagnostic laparotomy

This is a scenario of ruptured ectopic pregnancy and is the only possible answer. It is the only life-threatening, gynaecological emergency that requires immediate surgery.

13   D: Diagnostic laparoscopy and tubal dye test

The symptoms described here by the patient point towards endometriosis. Although both transvaginal Hycosy (hysterosalpingo contrast sonography) and HSG (hysterosalpingogram) help in diagnosing tubal and other uterine structural problems, they will not be able to assess the pelvis to diagnose endometriosis. Hence, it may be worthwhile to first think of the disease and then work out the best diagnostic modality in the given scenario.

14   I: Serum LH and serum FSH

This is because you suspect premature ovarian failure from her symptoms.

15   A: Cervical punch biopsy

This is obviously a case of suspected cervical malignancy that needs to be ruled out by tissue biopsy. The fact that the patient is an asylum seeker means she is not in the National Cervical Screening Programme.

Theme: Pelvic pain

16   G: Pyelonephritis

Loin pain and tenderness with fever and systemic upset suggest extension of the infection to the pelvis and kidney, known as 'pyelitis' or 'pyelonephritis'.

17   D: Diverticulitis
The fibroids are a red herring here. The symptoms are classic of acute diverticulitis.

18   H: Red degeneration of fibroid
The symphysis fundal height is much greater than the weeks of gestation and hence this is the most probable diagnosis. Red degeneration is seen only in pregnancy when there is ischaemic degeneration of the fibroid. There is not enough blood supply to sustain the growth of the fibroid.

19   A: Acute PID
Breakthrough bleeding in young pill users is often associated with pelvic inflammatory disease (PID). The other symptoms and clinical findings make the diagnosis very easy.

20   F: Endometriosis
Endometriotic ovarian cysts are referred to as 'endometriomas' or 'chocolate cysts'.

Theme: **Contraception**

21   C: Dianette®
Dianette® is the trade name for co-cyprindiol, which is a mixture of cyproterone acetate and ethinylestradiol in the mass proportions of 2000 parts to 35 parts, respectively. This is an anti-androgen and reduces acne by decreasing the sebum secretion under androgen control. Dianette® is the only licensed drug for acne and hirsutism in the UK. It is ideal for people who need contraception for whom acne is also a problem.

22   K: Progesterone-only pill
POP does not affect the volume of breast milk and provides 99% contraceptive efficacy when breast-feeding. The lactational amenorrhoea method (LAM) cannot be considered when the patient is not fully breast-feeding. Women may be advised that if they are less than 6 months' postpartum, amenorrhoeic and fully breast-feeding (no other liquids or solids given), the LAM is over 98% effective in preventing pregnancy.

23   G: Intrauterine copper device

A copper intrauterine contraceptive device (IUCD) can be inserted up to 5 days following unprotected intercourse, whereas the first dose of the morning-after pill must be taken within 72 hours of unprotected intercourse. Taking the first dose of levonorgestrel as soon as possible increases the efficacy. The dose is repeated 12 hours after the first tablet.

24   J: Mirena® coil

Considering the patient's age, her high BMI and menstrual problem this seems the best option. The Mirena® coil is a progesterone-only intrauterine system that releases 20 μg of levonorgestrel directly into the uterine cavity every 24 hours. It acts by preventing endometrial proliferation and is very effective in controlling menorrhagia.

25   E: Implanon®

This patient has a problem with contraceptive compliance and needs reliable long-term contraception. Taking into consideration that this patient has had STIs in the past, she would not be suitable for IUCDs. Although you can consider condoms, her history of poor compliance with the pill and injections and also the poor efficacy of condoms will not make these an ideal choice for her. Implanon® is an implant containing a progesterone contraceptive. It contains etonogestrel, is subdermally implanted and is effective for 3 years. It also has a very low Pearl Index (ie the measure of contraceptive efficacy expressed in 100 women-reproductive years).

Theme: Infertility/assisted reproductive technology

26   F: IVF with ICSI (*in vitro* fertilisation with intracytoplasmic sperm injection)

This is a difficult theme as infertility is not the forte of most people. It is important to try and identify whether it is the man, woman, or both, with the problem. Once you have done that then you can work out which is the best technique to overcome the problem. In this case there are both male (low count with poor motility) and female (poor quality eggs associated with an age of more than 35) factors involved, which are best overcome by this technique.

27 C: IUI (intrauterine insemination)

There is a male factor problem here. Hypospadias is a congenital defect where the urethra opens on the underside of the penis instead of the tip, hence there is an anatomical difficulty in the sperm reaching the egg. This can be overcome by IUI.

28 H: Ovulation induction with follicular tracking

This is the first-line medical management for women with anovulatory cycles. Some patients with polycystic ovarian syndrome (PCOS) who are refractory to ovulation induction can opt for surgical management in the form of laparoscopic multiple-diathermy punctures of the ovary.

29 D: IVF

This is fairly straightforward as the absence of tubes rules out the other options like GIFT/ZIFT. Considering the fact that she has conceived twice in the past rules out male factor subfertility.

30 I: Surrogacy

The patient, having had a hysterectomy, has lost her uterus and hence will be unable to bear any pregnancy. Thus they will need a donor uterus to bear their pregnancy, which can be provided by a surrogate mother. Once they have had a successful IVF cycle with the host egg and sperm, the embryos will then be transferred into the surrogate mother's uterus.

Theme: Sexually transmitted infections (STIs)

31 A: Chancroid

Chancroid, or soft chancre, is an acute STI, caused by *Haemophilus ducreyi*, which is endemic in parts of Asia and Africa. This is a painful chancre when compared to syphilitic or LGV (lymphogranuloma venereum) ulcers, which are painless.

32 G: Herpes simplex

Genital herpes is caused by the herpes simplex virus. Type 1 is responsible for oral herpes or cold sores and type 2 for genital herpes. However, with more people having oral sex, the differentiation is difficult.

33 I: HIV

Oral candidiasis is one of the opportunistic infections found in immunosuppressed HIV patients. Kaposi's sarcoma is a cutaneous manifestation of AIDS, initially caused by proliferation of small blood vessels in the dermis. Later, nodules are formed with proliferating spindle cells and intradermal haemorrhage and the deposition of haemosiderin.

34 C: Gonorrhoea

The symptoms are classic of gonococcal PID (pelvic inflammatory disease). The finding of a Bartholin's abscess is diagnostic. In the past, more than 50% of women in the reproductive age group with a Bartholin's abscess tested positive for gonorrhoea.

35 E: Hepatitis B

The viral markers make the diagnosis easy. The presence of anti-HBe gives a picture of chronic hepatitis B infection. Both hepatitis B and C can be contracted by intravenous drug users.

Theme: Vaginal discharge

36 K: Vulvovaginitis

This is the commonest gynaecological problem in the prepubertal age group. Due to low levels of oestrogen between birth and puberty, the vaginal mucosa is thin and alkaline, making it less resistant to bacteria. Management takes the form of reassuring anxious parents, maintaining good hygiene and wearing cotton undergarments.

37 A: Atrophic vaginitis

This is a classic presentation that you see in the clinic. The dry, thin, atrophic vaginal mucosa rubs against the undergarments and causes bleeding and staining.

38 C: Candidiasis
This is a typical picture of vulval candidiasis and is treated with
Canesten® (clotrimazole) pessaries. In chronic candidiasis the
treatment is given 1 week before and after menstruation and
continued for 6 months. It is also important to treat the partner
to eliminate re-infection.

39 E: Ectropion
This is the commonest cause of a clear, non-itchy vaginal
discharge. This is common among pill users as it induces
columnar epithelium to spread over the transformation zone.
Columnar epithelium is secretory.

40 J: *Trichomonas vaginalis* (TV)
This is a typical discharge found in TV infections. On
per-speculum examination the cervix is seen to have multiple
small haemorrhagic areas, which lead to the description
'strawberry cervix'. Metronidazole 400 mg, twice/thrice a day for
7 days is the treatment of choice.

Theme: Endocrine disorders

41 A: Congenital adrenal hyperplasia (CAH)
This is an autosomal recessive disorder caused by deficiency of
one of the enzymes in the cortisol synthesis pathway. Hence,
cortisol secretion is reduced, resulting in an increased feedback
and increased secretion of ACTH. This in turn leads to diversion
of the pathway into the production of androgenic steroid
hormones. It can also be associated with aldosterone suppression,
causing hypoadrenalism and salt-wasting. Increased androgen
production leads to signs of virilisation.

42 C: Graves' disease
This form of autoimmune thyroiditis is associated with
thyrotoxicosis. Eye signs are an important feature. It can also be
associated with other autoimmune disorders like pernicious
anaemia and myasthenia gravis.

43 B: Craniopharyngioma
The visual symptoms are due to compression of the optic chiasma

by the tumour. The other features are due to hypopituitarism.

44   E: Hypogonadotrophic hypogonadism (Kallmann's syndrome)

This is an isolated deficiency of LHRH (luteinising hormone-releasing hormone) or LH/FSH. It is often associated with anosmia, cleft palate, renal abnormalities and cerebral abnormalities such as colour blindness. It is usually familial and shows an X-linked inheritance pattern.

45   H: Polycystic ovarian syndrome (PCOS)

PCOS is associated with a mild elevation of serum prolactin (rarely going beyond 1500 IU) due to the altered pituitary-ovarian axis.

Theme: Chromosomal abnormalities

These are all questions on factual knowledge and you need to read your textbooks to learn about these conditions.

46   I: Patau's syndrome

Also known as trisomy 13, the incidence of this syndrome is 1:5000. It can be diagnosed prenatally by amniocentesis or by chorionic villus sampling. Babies rarely survive for more than a few weeks.

47   F: Huntington's disease

This autosomal dominant, inevitably fatal disease, with a prevalence of 1:20,000, is associated with progressive chorea and dementia in middle age. There is cerebral atrophy, with a marked reduction in the number of neurones in the caudate nucleus and putamen of the brain. In addition, there is an associated decrease in the levels of neurotransmitters.

48   J: Sickle cell disease

This results from a single base mutation of adenine to thymine that produces a substitution of valine for glutamine at the sixth codon of the β-globin chain. If this is homozygous then the genes on both chromosomes are affected, whereas only one chromosome carries the affected gene in heterozygotes. This disease is mainly prevalent in Africa, but is also reported in the Indian subcontinent, the Middle East and southern Europe.

49 G: Klinefelter's syndrome
This chromosomal abnormality (47,XXY) affects about 1:1000 males. Associated with dysgenesis of the seminiferous tubules and an absence of Leydig cells, it results in congenital male hypogonadism.

50 C: Fragile X syndrome
This sex-linked chromosomal disorder is due to an abnormality in the X chromosome. Both males and females can inherit this abnormal chromosome.

Theme: **Vulval disorders**

51 B: Carcinoma of the vulva
The presence of such a characteristic ulcer with lymphadenopathy is diagnostic of a cancerous lesion.

52 H: Varicose veins
Vulval varicosity is worsened in pregnancy due to the pressure of the gravid uterus obstructing venous drainage from the lower extremity.

53 E: Leucoplakia
The only sure way to differentiate this from lichen sclerosis is by tissue biopsy. On clinical examination lichen sclerosis initially appear purplish and then turns white, with a shiny, thin skin.

54 K: Vulval wart
Vulval warts are caused by the human papillomavirus (HPV). They become more florid in immunosuppressed conditions like pregnancy. HPV-18 and -33 have been implicated in cervical intraepithelial neoplasia. It is sexually transmitted and both partners need to be treated if present in both.

55 G: Sebaceous cyst
This is a typical presentation and the patient is often referred by the GP with a diagnosis of Bartholin's abscess.

Theme: Gynaecological surgery

56   E: Manchester's operation
A modified form of this operation is also known as 'Fothergill's operation'.

57   F: Marsupialisation
This is the surgical treatment for Bartholin's abscess. By everting the cyst wall margins you are trying to prevent its recurrence.

58   H: Shirodkar's suture
This can be differentiated from McDonald's suture when you put purse-string sutures around the cervix without deflecting the bladder.

59   K: Zacharin procedure
This surgical procedure corrects the anatomical defect in the levator hiatus in patients who have a persistent vault prolapse after hysterectomy. This combined abdominal and vaginal procedure has a good outcome overall.

60   J: Wertheim's surgery
This is the surgery for stage I and stage IIA cancer of the cervix.

Theme: Abdominal swellings

61   F: Ovarian hyperstimulation syndrome (OHSS)
This is caused by a sudden excessive multiplication of ovarian follicles in response to follicle-stimulating drugs. This results in diffuse abdominal pain and cystic enlargement of the ovaries. It is classified into mild, moderate and severe, depending on the size of the ovaries and the presence of other factors like ascites and deranged blood count, liver function tests and U&E. In some cases it can be associated with pleural and pericardial effusions. Management depends on careful fluid replacement, depending on the haematocrit, WCC, etc. It is important to ensure thromboprophylactic measures, like anti-embolic stockings and low-dose heparin, are taken as these patients are at a higher risk of thrombosis due to reduced intravascular volume. Severe cases need management in the ITU and draining of ascites and pleural effusions for symptomatic relief.

62   H: Ovarian teratoma
These are germ-cell tumours and have an embryonic origin. They are common in young women, associated with torsion and in about 20% of the cases are bilateral.

63   A: Adenomyosis
Endometriosis of the uterine musculature is called 'adenomyosis'. Apart from an enlarged uterus there is no other clinical diagnostic feature. Diagnosis is based on the symptoms of cyclical pain with the menses. Medical treatment involves suppression of ovulation, whereas surgical management encompasses endometrial ablation, resection and, finally, hysterectomy.

64   J: Strangulated hernia
The treatment is immediate laparotomy.

65   D: Haematometra
The aetiology for this is an imperforate hymen. Although a rare clinical finding, it can catch you off guard. It is always associated with primary amenorrhoea and the patient gives a history of monthly abdominal pain and swelling. On examination you find the hymen bulging out like a membrane under the pressure of the collected blood (haematocolpos). Treatment is incision and drainage of the collected blood. Haematometra and pyometra can also occur when the cervical canal is blocked by a growth in cases of frank cervical malignancy.

Theme: **Obstetric emergencies**

66   H: Shoulder dystocia
This is a classic description of the situation when the head comes out but the shoulders get stuck. The incidence of this obstetric emergency is between 0.15% and 1.7%. Although fetal macrosomia is an important risk factor, more than half the incidence of shoulder dystocia is reported among babies weighing less than 4 kg. The management involves manoeuvres to deliver the shoulders in addition to gentle traction downwards (to disimpact the shoulders) and an episiotomy.

67 E: Perineal trauma

The clinical findings of a hard and contracted uterus rule out an atonic postpartum haemorrhage (PPH).

68 K: Uterine rupture

The incidence of scar dehiscence is about 0.5% in women who go into spontaneous labour with a history of a previous Caesarean section. This risk is greatly increased if labour is induced or augmented with oxytocics or prostaglandins. The management of scar rupture is a 'crash Caesarean section'. It is associated with high fetal morbidity and mortality, and only a high index of suspicion and prompt action improves the outcome. A constant complaint of abdominal pain (even when the uterus is relaxed), sudden collapse and abdominal palpation of fetal parts are other signs and symptoms associated with this obstetric emergency.

69 G: Pulmonary embolism

Pregnancy, pelvic surgery and immobilisation increase the risk of these patients developing a pulmonary embolism and DVT (deep vein thrombosis). Always have this diagnosis at the back of your mind when dealing with any patient with unexplained postoperative collapse.

70 J: Uterine inversion

Although uncommon, uterine inversion is a life-threatening complication in the third stage of labour. Poor management of the third stage of labour, including pulling on an unseparated placenta, fundal pressure to deliver the placenta and manual removal of the placenta have all been implicated. Management involves immediate replacement of the uterus and active resuscitation.

Theme: Breast disorders

71 G: Fibroadenoma

These are no longer thought to be benign breast tumours and are instead regarded as aberrations in breast development. However, you still need to investigate and reach your diagnosis based on a combination of scan and FNAC (fine-needle aspiration cytology) findings.

72   D: Breast cancer

This is clearly a case of breast cancer. Skin dimpling is caused by local infiltration of malignancy and *peau d'orange* is due to lymphatic oedema. Both these signs are suggestive of locally advanced cancer.

73   E: Duct ectasia

This condition is age-related and as women age the ducts shorten and dilate, resulting in inversion of the nipple. This should be differentiated from that seen in malignant conditions where the nipple appears retracted and pulled in.

74   C: Breast abscess

The mention of swelling clearly helps in making the diagnosis. Non-lactational breast abscesses are becoming more common and the causative organisms are usually a *Staphylococcus* and/or other anaerobes.

75   J: Lipoma

These are benign fatty lumps that occur in any part of the body where fat can expand.

Theme: High-risk pregnancy

76   C: Intravenous antibiotics

This woman is in established labour and needs immediate antibiotic prophylaxis against GBS. This is to prevent the transfer of infection from mother to the baby as it passes through the birth canal. GBS infections notoriously cause early-onset neonatal septicaemia. Presently, any woman who is tested positive for GBS during the antenatal period, or at any time in their reproductive lifespan, needs antibiotic prophylaxis against GBS during labour. In order to familiarise yourself with obstetric practices in the UK you can refer to the RCOG website (*www.rcog.org.uk*).

77   B: Immediate delivery

This seems the most logical management as the pregnancy is at 35 weeks and the risk of RDS due to lung immaturity is much reduced at this gestation. This is a case of gross IUGR (intrauterine growth retardation) and the baby is at a high risk of sudden intrauterine death (IUD).

78 I: Serial cervical-length assessment by transvaginal scan

Although you might be tempted to put in a cervical suture, careful analysis of the patient's history of presentation directs you to the fact that her last premature delivery was probably due to an infection rather than to an incompetent cervix. The fact that she came in with pain and contractions points towards infection being the underlying cause.

79 E: Low-dose aspirin

Lupus anticoagulant and anticardiolipin antibody together are features of the antiphospholipid syndrome (APS). Diagnosis is made when the patient has one of the clinical features (history of fetal loss, thrombosis, autoimmune thrombocytopenia, etc) and lupus anticoagulant or medium to high titres of IgG anticardiolipin antibodies, or both. In this case the patient has antiphospholipid antibodies without APS and low-dose aspirin is the best treatment option. Women with symptomatic APS need to be on prophylactic doses of heparin during pregnancy.

80 H: Screening for bacterial vaginosis

Bacterial vaginosis accounts for about 30% of the cases of preterm deliveries. It is one of the preventable causes and screening of high-risk women can reduce its impact. Screening involves taking a high vaginal swab (HVS) at the booking visit and repeating it at every antenatal visit until delivery. If bacterial vaginosis is picked up on an HVS it is treated with metronidazole, 400 mg three times each day for 5 days.

81 B: Cefalexin

This is the most commonly used broad-spectrum antibiotic in pregnancy for treating suspected UTIs. This is safe and usually covers the most common organisms responsible for urinary tract infection in pregnancy. Both tetracyclines and trimethoprim are teratogenic and are not used in pregnancy.

82 G: Methyldopa

This is the most commonly used and the safest antihypertensive used in pregnancy. Atenolol is not usually used due to the risk of causing intrauterine growth retardation.

83 H: Misoprostol per rectum

Misoprostol, an prostaglandin E1 analogue, has recently been found to be very effective in treating PPH via the rectal route when compared with conventional oxytocics. However, there still much ongoing debate regarding its efficacy. Large ongoing studies are trying to determine its true effectiveness.

84 F: Methotrexate

The criteria for offering medical management for ectopic pregnancy in a haemodynamically stable patient includes: an adnexal or tubal mass with a diameter of less than 3 cm; an ovary seen to be separate from the mass; no intraperitoneal blood or fetal heart seen; and an initial βHCG of $<$ 2000 IU. Methotrexate, a folic acid antagonist; is given intramuscularly in a single dose regime of 50 mg/m^2 using a chemotherapy surface area/height/weight chart.

85 E: Magnesium sulphate

The recent Magpie trial has established magnesium sulphate as the drug of choice in managing eclampsia and also that it is beneficial in preventing impending eclampsia. It acts as a vasodilator and as a membrane stabiliser. It also acts as a central anticonvulsant by blocking the *N*-methyl-*d*-aspartate receptor in the hippocampus and reduces the incidence of recurrent convulsions. It reduces maternal mortality and the need for ventilatory support and admission to ITU. Its smooth muscle relaxant effect causes respiratory depression, and other side-effects include diplopia, flushes, slurred speech, loss of patellar reflexes and paralysis due to toxicity at the neuromuscular junction.

Obstetrics and Gynaecology SBAs

1 A 50-year-old woman comes to the menopause clinic requesting advice about HRT. She is concerned about her risk of developing osteoporosis as both her mother and sister suffered pelvic fractures due to osteoporosis after the menopause.

What is the SINGLE best test that will give an estimation of her risk of developing osteoporosis?

A   Dual-energy X-ray absorptiometry (DEXA)
B   MRI of the pelvis
C   Pelvic X-ray
D   Serum alkaline phosphatase
E   Serum calcium

2 A 48-year-old woman comes to the menopausal clinic complaining of severe vasomotor symptoms of hot flushes and night sweats. She is extremely anxious about going on HRT as she had a DVT when she was pregnant, 20 years ago. However, she has been fine ever since and has required no long-term treatment. She has read in the papers that HRT increases the risk of getting a clot.

What is the SINGLE best form of HRT for her?

A   Oral continuous combined HRT
B   Oral sequential combined HRT
C   Raloxifene
D   Tibolone
E   Transdermal combined HRT patches

3 A 26-year-old woman, who is 28 weeks' pregnant, complains of breathlessness during a routine antenatal check-up. On clinical examination you notice everything to be normal apart from the fact that she is slightly hyperventilating.

Which ONE of the following findings would you be surprised to encounter during a normal pregnancy?

A   Decrease in the serum ferritin level
B   Increase in cardiac output
C   Increase in glomerular filtration rate (GFR)
D   Increase in the levels of clotting factors VII, VIII and IX
E   Increase in total lung capacity

4 An anxious 28-weeks pregnant woman comes to see you, her GP, with a history of indirect exposure to chickenpox. While taking a history you gather that one of her neighbour's children has chickenpox. The patient is not sure whether she had chickenpox as a child.

What is the SINGLE best management for this patient?

A   Aciclovir
B   Check for serum varicella zoster IgG (VZIgG)
C   Immunoglobulins and aciclovir
D   Termination of pregnancy
E   Varicella zoster vaccination

5 A 23-year-old known IDDM patient comes to your clinic for pre-pregnancy counselling with regard to her glycaemic control and the right time for her to try for a baby.

Which ONE of the following is the best test that will help you to advise the patient?

A HbA_{1C}
B   1-hour GTT
C   2-hour GTT
D   Random blood sugar
E   Sugar series

6 A 37-year-old primigravida, 10 weeks' pregnant, comes to your antenatal clinic for counselling about Down's syndrome screening as her brother has Down's syndrome. After discussing the various tests with her, she decides to opt for the earliest possible diagnostic test that will tell her whether this is a Down's pregnancy or not.

Which SINGLE test are you most likely to advise her to have?

A   Amniocentesis   D   Nuchal translucency test
B   Anomaly scan   E   Triple blood test
C   Chorionic villus sampling (CVS)

7 A 26-year-old woman and her 28-year-old partner come to the GP surgery complaining of primary infertility for 2 years. She gives a history of irregular menstrual cycles.

What is the SINGLE best test to see whether she is ovulating or not?

A   Basal body temperature estimation
B   Cervical fern test
C   Day-2 LH and FSH
D   Day-21 progesterone level
E   Endometrial biopsy

Obstetrics and Gynaecology SBAs – Answers

1 A: DEXA

After the menopause the lack of oestrogen causes bone loss and 1 in 2 women have a risk of developing an osteoporotic fracture by the age of 70 years. Immobility and lack of exercise in the later years adds to the risk. There may be a genetic predisposition as some women are 'fast bone losers'. An at-risk woman should be given a DEXA scan to measure her bone density and then, by comparing her bone density with that of her peer group, her subsequent fracture risk can be estimated.

2 E: Transdermal combined HRT patches

Although the patient had a DVT in the past, this seems to have been related to her pregnancy. The transdermal route seems to be the best option as it bypasses the enterohepatic circulation, and hence reduces the effect on the hepatic clotting system. You need to ensure that a woman with a previous history of DVT or PE has been screened for thrombophilia and has a normal clotting profile. The risk in the general population of getting a clot is 1 in 10,000 per year, which increases to 3 in 10,000 for those on HRT.

3 E: Increase in total lung capacity

Total lung capacity is decreased in pregnancy by about 200 ml. This is because the residual volume is reduced by 200 ml, secondary to the large intra-abdominal swelling in pregnancy.

4 B: Check for serum varicella zoster IgG (VZIgG)

If a susceptible mother is exposed to a source of varicella zoster virus, then this may result in a primary varicella infection in pregnancy. Maternal varicella in the first 20 weeks of pregnancy carries a 1–2% risk of developing varicella embryopathy syndrome in the fetus. The consequences of fetal varicella syndrome include scarring of the skin, hypoplasia of limbs and chorioretinitis. Adult varicella can cause pnuemonitis as a serious complication.

Neonatal varicella occurs when the mother has chickenpox in late pregnancy and the interval between the mother developing the rash and the delivery of the baby is not sufficient for the mother to pass on protective antibodies to the fetus *in utero*.

5   A: HbA$_{1C}$

This test measures the average blood glucose concentration over the lifespan of a haemoglobin molecule, which is approximately 6 weeks. Levels below 6% are considered to be a reflection of good glycaemic control and the patient can start trying for a baby at this stage, with folic acid supplementation. As diabetic mothers have an increased risk of having babies with neural tube defects, folic acid supplementation is one of the preventive measures.

6   C: Chorionic villus sampling

CVS is the diagnostic procedure for karyotyping in the first trimester. The disadvantage of this procedure is its higher incidence of procedure-related miscarriage rates. In addition, the rate of mosaicism is higher with CVS, necessitating a subsequent amniocentesis in a small proportion of pregnancies.

7   D: Day-21 progesterone level

This is the easiest test to check her ovulatory status. If D21 progesterone results are more than 30 nmol/l in two cycles, then the patient is ovulating.

Paediatrics

Chapter contributed by
Dr Abanti Paul MBBS DCH DRCOG MRCGP

Paediatric EMQs

Theme: **Diagnosis of normal developmental milestones**

Options

A	6 weeks	G	12 months
B	3 months	H	15 months
C	4 months	I	18 months
D	6 months	J	24 months
E	8 months	K	36 months
F	10 months	L	40 months

Instructions

For each of the children described below choose the SINGLE most appropriate milestone age from the list of options above. Each option may be used once, more than once or not at all.

1 Abbie's head does not fall back when her mother pulls her from a lying to a sitting position. ☐

2 Bobby starts cruising around the furniture and grasps objects between his thumb and forefinger. ☐

3 John starts walking alone and builds a tower with three cubes. *18 mo* ☐

4 Lucy starts riding a tricycle, builds a tower with 10 cubes and copies a circle. ☐

5 Rob says 'mama' and 'dada', and drinks from a cup. ☐

Theme: **Common skin conditions in childhood**

Options

A   Eczema
B   Erythema multiforme
C   Henoch–Schönlein purpura
D   Impetigo

E   Molluscum contagiosum
F   Pityriasis rosea
G   Psoriasis
H   Scabies

Instructions

For each of the patients described below choose the SINGLE most appropriate diagnosis from the list of options above. Each option may be used once, more than once or not at all.

6 A 4-year-old boy had a cough a week ago. He now presents with abdominal pain and rashes on his buttocks and the extensor surfaces of his legs. ☐

7 A 14-year-old boy presents with extensive pink macules over his chest and back. He recalls that the big macule on the left side of his chest was the first to appear. ☐

8 A 3-year-old child complains of severe itching at night. On examination she has tiny papules and vesicles between her fingers and on her wrist. ☐

9 A 12-year-old girl presents with plaques over her elbows and the back of her ears. She also complains of pain in the small joints of her hand. On examination her nails are pitted. ☐

10 A 4-year-old boy has recently been going for swimming lessons. His mother notices that he has small pearly lesions on his tummy. ☐

Theme: **Children with fits**

Options

A	Absences	E	Neurofibromatosis
B	Cerebral palsy	F	Sturge–Weber syndrome
C	Febrile convulsions	G	Tuberous sclerosis A
D	Grand mal epilepsy	H	Waardenburg's syndrome

Instructions

For each of the patients described below choose the SINGLE most appropriate diagnosis from the list of options above. Each option may be used once, more than once or not at all.

11 Rob is now 6 months old. His mother is worried that he still can't hold his head up, is difficult to feed and feels floppy, like a rag doll.

12 A 4-year-old child is referred to you with an acneiform rash over her nose and cheeks, delayed milestones and frequent fits. On examination she has fibromas under her nails.

13 An 11-year-old boy with learning difficulties is referred to you because of frequent fits. On examination he has freckles in his axillas.

14 A 4-year-old child was born with a red discoloration of the right side of her face. She presents with fits and weakness of her right arm and leg.

15 A 9-month-old febrile child presents with sudden-onset jerking of all four limbs and unresponsiveness. This lasts for 2 minutes and the child is drowsy afterwards.

Theme: **Children with coughs**

Options

H influenza

A	Acute epiglottitis *thumb print*	F	Diphtheria
B	Angio-oedema	G	Foreign-body inhalation
C	Asthma	H	Pertussis
D	Bronchiolitis *RSV*	I	Retropharyngeal abscess
E	Cystic fibrosis	J	Viral croup *steeple sign*

parainfluenza   *on CXR*

Instructions

For each of the patients described below choose the SINGLE most appropriate diagnosis from the list of options above. Each option may be used once, more than once or not at all.

16 A 2-year-old boy with a history of fever and running nose for 2 days is brought to A&E at night with a barking cough and stridor. ☐

17 A 3-year-old child with a history of a raised temperature and coryza for the last 2–3 days develops a paroxysmal spasmodic cough followed by inspiratory whoops. ☐

18 A 6-month-old baby is brought to the paediatric day unit with dry cough, difficulty in feeding and breathlessness (it is winter). On examination her chest is hyperinflated, with fine crackles. ☐

19 A 5-year-old girl presents with a severe sore throat, difficulty in breathing, and drooling of saliva. The child is sitting upright with her mouth wide open. *intubate + IV antibiotics* ☐

20 A 6-year-old boy presents with a troublesome nocturnal cough. He gets breathless after sports and his brother suffers from eczema. ☐

21 A 3-year-old child is referred because of recurrent chest infections and poor weight gain in spite of a voracious appetite. On examination he has nasal polyps. ☐

Theme: **Abdominal pain**

Options

A   Abdominal migraine
B   Acute appendicitis
C   Constipation
D   Diabetic ketoacidosis
E   Hirschsprung's disease
F   Infantile colic
G   Intussusception

H   Irritable bowel syndrome
I   Mesenteric adenitis
J   Pancreatitis
K   Peritonitis
L   Renal calculus
M   Torsion of the testis

Instructions

For each of the patients described below choose the SINGLE most appropriate diagnosis from the list of options above. Each option may be used once, more than once or not at all.

22 A 3-month-old child is brought with paroxysmal inconsolable crying, with her legs drawn up, in the evenings.

23 A 5-year-old boy with a history of cough and swollen neck glands, presents with abdominal pain. On examination his abdomen is soft, but there is no guarding, and he is tender in the right iliac fossa.

24 A 2-year-old boy is brought with a sudden-onset colicky pain. He looks pale, draws up his legs during a pain episode and passes a red, jelly-like stool.

25 A 4-year-old boy with anorexia, vomiting and a high temperature presents with abdominal pain that initially is central, then moves to the right iliac fossa.

26 A 7-year-old boy presents with paroxysmal abdominal pain with facial pallor; he is otherwise well. There is a family history of migraine.

27 An 8-year-old boy complains that he has had an intermittent colicky abdominal pain and bloated feeling for months. The pain is relieved by defecation; sometimes his stools are normal and sometimes he is constipated.

Theme: **Diarrhoea**

Options

A   Coeliac disease
B   Crohn's disease
C   Milk intolerance

D   Toddler's diarrhoea
E   Ulcerative colitis
F   Viral gastroenteritis

Instructions

For each of the patients described below choose the SINGLE most appropriate diagnosis from the list of options above. Each option may be used once, more than once or not at all.

28 An 18-month-old child is brought in irritable, with persistent diarrhoea, abdominal distension and wasting of the buttocks. ☐

29 A 4-year-old boy presents with altered bowel motions and stools containing undigested vegetables. Otherwise the child is well and thriving. ☐

30 A 14-year-old girl presents with intermittent fever, diarrhoea and joint pain, On examination she has ulcers in her mouth. Her periods have not yet started and she has poor breast development. ☐

31 A 2-month-old baby, just started being bottle-fed, presents with protracted diarrhoea and poor weight gain. She also suffers from eczema.   *IgA def.* ☐

Theme: **Painful limbs in children**

Options

A	Chondromalacia patellae	F	Perthes disease
B	Juvenile idiopathic arthritis	G	Septic arthritis
C	Leukaemia	H	Slipped femoral epiphysis
D	Non-accidental injury	I	Transient synovitis *2 –12 y/o*
E	Osgood–Schlatter disease	J	Trauma

10 – 17 yr
overuse

Instructions

*For each of the patients described below choose the SINGLE most
appropriate diagnosis from the list of options above. Each option may be
used once, more than once or not at all.*

32 A 4-year-old boy presents complaining of pain in his right hip
following a viral illness, no pain at rest, but with decreased
abduction. The child is afebrile. His WCC is normal, as is his
CRP. ☐

33 A 14-year-old football player complains of pain in his right
knee. On examination there is pain and tenderness over the
tibial tubercle. ☐

34 A 10-year-old boy complains of pain in his left hip, which
started after minor trauma. There is restricted abduction and
internal rotation. He is obese. ☐

35 A 2-year-old boy presents with a high temperature. He is unwell
and complaining of severe pain. There is pain at rest and no
movement at his right hip. His WCC and CRP are raised. ☐

36 A 4-week-old baby is brought to A&E with a swollen left shin.
Her parents say she hurt herself when she rolled off the bed. ☐

Theme: **Investigations for failure to thrive**

Options

A	Acute-phase reactant	F	Ferritin
B	Anti-endomysial and antigliadin antibodies	G	Immunoglobulins
		H	Liver function tests
C	Chest X-ray and sweat test	I	Plasma creatinine and electrolytes
D	Chromosomal analysis	J	Stool microscopy and culture
E	FBC, WCC	K	Thyroid function tests

Instructions

For each of the diagnoses described below choose the SINGLE most appropriate investigation from the list of options above. Each option may be used once, more than once or not at all.

37 Cystic fibrosis ☐

38 Intestinal infection ☐

39 Turner's syndrome ☐

40 Coeliac disease ☐

41 Iron deficiency anaemia ☐

42 Crohn's disease ☐

43 Hypothyroidism ☐

Theme: **Respiratory distress in the newborn**

Options

A	Diaphragmatic hernia	E	Pneumothorax
B	Meconium aspiration	F	Pulmonary haemorrhage
C	Milk aspiration	G	Pulmonary hypoplasia
D	Pneumonia	H	Transient tachypnoea

Instructions

For each of the patients described below choose the SINGLE most appropriate diagnosis from the list of options above. Each option may be used once, more than once or not at all.

44 A baby has been born at 42 weeks' gestation with respiratory distress. The chest X-ray shows an over-inflated chest with patches of consolidation and collapse. ☐

45 A baby has been born with respiratory distress. His mother is pyrexial and her membranes ruptured 48 hours before giving birth. ☐

46 A preterm baby has become increasingly breathless after 24 hours of being on a ventilator. ☐

47 A baby develops respiratory distress on feeding. On examination the child has a cleft palate. ☐

48 A child born by Caesarean section is in respiratory distress. A chest X-ray shows fluid in the horizontal fissure, but the breathlessness settles within the first day of life. ☐

49 A baby has been born with respiratory distress and is not responding to resuscitation. On examination the apex beat and heart sounds are displaced to the right side of its chest. ☐

Theme: **Screening tests**

Options

A   At 8 months of age
B   At school entry
C   Between a child's fourth and fifth birthdays
D   Day 5–6 of life
E   In primary school
F   In secondary school
G   Soon after birth
H   Within the first week of life

Instructions

For each of the tests described below choose the SINGLE most appropriate time for screening from the list of options above. Each option may be used once, more than once or not at all.

50 Orthoptist assessment of a child's vision.

51 General physical examination with emphasis on eyes, heart and hips.

52 Blood spot test for hypothyroidism and phenylketonuria.

53 Height and weight measurements and a sweep test for hearing.

54 Infant distraction test which is being done presently, but note that this will soon be phased out.

55 Automated hearing screen, which is recommended to be phased in by 2005.

Theme: **Teratogenic drugs**

Options

A	Combined oral contraceptive pill	F	Progestogens
B	Diethylstilbestrol	G	Propylthiouracil
C	Digoxin	H	Tetracycline
D	Lithium	I	Thalidomide
E	Phenytoin	J	Warfarin

Instructions

For each of the adverse effects described below choose the SINGLE most likely maternal medication taken during pregnancy from the list of options above. Each option may be used once, more than once or not at all.

56 Children may have discoloured teeth. □

57 A high dose of this drug is associated with clear-cell vaginal adenocarcinoma and urogenital abnormality in the child. □

58 Babies are born with a small head size and a hypoplastic nose. □

59 Babies born to mothers taking this medication have hypoplastic nails and a cleft palate. □

60 Babies are born with short limbs and/or missing limbs. □

Paediatric EMQs – Answers

Theme: Diagnosis of normal developmental milestones

1 C: 4 months

2 F: 10 months

3 I: 18 months

4 K: 36 months

5 G: 12 months

At 4 months a baby should be able to hold its head straight when pulled to a sitting position; at 6 months sit without support with a round back; at 8 months sit with a straight back.

At 9 months the baby should be crawling; at 10 months cruising around furniture; by 1 year walking with one hand held; by 18 months walking without support and building tower of 3 blocks; and by 3 years the toddler should be able to ride a tricycle.

Children should be able to drink from a cup at 12 months and feed themselves with a spoon at 18 months.

NB. It is essential to learn a list of developmental milestones from any paediatric textbook. Remember the areas of development: gross motor, fine motor and vision, speech and hearing, social.

Theme: Common skin conditions in childhood

6 C: Henoch-Schönlein purpura

HSP is a self-limiting vasculitis that occurs between the ages of 3 and 10 years, peaks during winter months and is preceded by a respiratory infection. Affected children often have a fever, but the most obvious feature is the rash, which is symmetrically distributed over the buttocks and extensor surfaces of the arms,

legs and ankles. Joints are affected, particularly those of the knee
and ankle. Many children experience a colicky abdominal pain,
which responds to steroid treatment. Intussusception can occur.
Renal involvement is common: 80% of patients develop a
macroscopic or microscopic haematuria, or mild proteinuria.
Most cases of haematuria resolve spontaneously. Heavy
proteinuria may indicate a rapidly progressive
glomerulonephritis, often with a nephritic phase. A small number
of patients develop acute renal failure and hypertension and
require dialysis.

7   F: Pityriasis rosea

This disease, affecting teenagers and young adults, is probably
caused by a virus. The herald patch is a 1–5-cm scaly lesion,
followed by the main eruption 2–3 weeks later. Common in
spring and autumn, it is often mistaken for ringworm. The rashes,
which resemble a fir tree, mainly appear over the trunk and
proximal limbs, especially on the back. It is a self-limiting
condition that resolves in 4–6 weeks.

8   H: Scabies

Scabies is caused by the *Sarcoptes scabiei* mite and is transmitted
by close contact. It typically affects the interdigital webs, axillas
and belt line, as well as around the nipples, penis, buttocks and
flexor surfaces of the wrists. Burrows, papules and vesicles are
found in these areas. These are particularly itchy at night and may
persist even after treatment for 4–6 weeks as scabies is due to
sensitisation. The whole family needs to be treated.

9   G: Psoriasis

Psoriasis with plaques and annular lesions is not common in
children. Fine pitting of the nails may be seen in chronic disease
but is uncommon in children. Occasionally, children may develop
arthropathy.

10   E: Molluscum contagiosum

This disease is caused by a DNA poxvirus and is commonly
spread by direct contact or fomites. It typically presents with
pearly umbilicated lesions anywhere on the body. Common
amongst children, especially those who are
immunocompromised. Children often contract the virus when

swimming in public swimming pools. It is infectious for as long as it is present but resolves spontaneously without treatment. Treatment is limited for cosmetic reasons.

Theme: Children with fits

11   B: Cerebral palsy
Cerebral palsy is a disorder of movement and posture caused by a non-progressive lesion of the motor pathways in a developing brain. The main causes are as follows:
- antenatal (80%): cerebral dysgenesis, cerebral malformation, congenital infection (rubella, toxoplasmosis, cytomegalovirus);
- intrapartum (10%): birth trauma and birth asphyxia
- postnatal (10%): meningitis, encephalitis, intraventricular haemorrhage, non-accidental injury, trauma to head, hydrocephalus and hyperbilirubinaemia.

Diagnosis is by clinical examination, with particular attention to assessment of posture, tone and observation of gait.

12   G: Tuberous sclerosis
This autosomal dominant condition may present with infantile spasm in infancy and epilepsy in later childhood. Common features are shagreen patches, ash-leaf macules, periungal fibromas and adenoma sebaceum in puberty.

13   E: Neurofibromatosis
Skin changes in neurofibromatosis include multiple skin nodules along the distribution of nerves, axillary freckling and more than five café-au-lait spots or brown macules, mainly over the trunk. Epilepsy and mental retardation occur in 10% of cases.

14   F: Sturge–Weber syndrome
This is a sporadic disorder with haemangiomatous facial lesions (port-wine stains) in the distribution of the trigeminal nerve, which is associated with a similar lesion intracranially. In the more severe form it may present with epilepsy, learning disabilities and hemiplegia.

15 C: Febrile convulsions

Febrile convulsions affect 3% of all children, commonly occurring between 6 months and 5 years of age. A seizure occurs early in a viral infection when the child's temperature is rising rapidly. The seizure lasts for 1–2 minutes and is generalised tonic or tonic-clonic in nature. In about 15% of cases, a seizure recurs during the same illness. The overall risk of a further febrile convulsion is 1 in 3. Febrile convulsions usually have a benign prognosis, but epilepsy subsequently develops in about 1% of cases.

Theme: **Children with coughs**

16 J: Viral croup

Viral croup is most often caused by the parainfluenza virus. It commonly occurs in children from 6 months to 6 years of age. Typical features are a barking cough, harsh stridor and hoarseness, usually preceded by fever and coryza. It often starts, and is worse, at night.

17 H: Pertussis

Pertussis is a highly infectious form of bronchitis caused by *Bordetella pertussis.* After 2–3 days of coryza, the child develops a characteristic paroxysmal or spasmodic cough followed by an inspiratory whoop (which gives pertussis its common name 'whooping cough'). The cough is worse at night and may be followed by vomiting. Epistaxis and subconjunctival haemorrhage may occur. Symptoms persist for 10–12 weeks.

18 D: Bronchiolitis

Bronchiolitis is the commonest serious respiratory infection of infancy. Caused by the respiratory syncytial virus in 80% of cases, it is common in the winter months. Coryzal symptoms precede a dry cough and increasing breathlessness. Wheeze is often present. Feeding difficulty is associated with dyspnoea.

19 A: Acute epiglottitis

Acute epiglottitis is a life-threatening emergency because of the respiratory obstruction. It is caused by *Haemophilus influenzae* type b. The disease is common in children between the ages of 1 and 6 years. Its onset is often very acute, with a high fever, a toxic-looking child, an intensely painful throat that stops the child from speaking and swallowing, and saliva that drools down the chin. Soft stridor is present. The child sits immobile and upright with an open mouth to optimise their airway.

20 C: Asthma

Asthma affects 10–15% of schoolchildren. In childhood it is twice as common in boys as in girls, but by adolescence the ratio is equal. Diagnosis is clinical and depends on a history of recurrent wheeze, cough and breathlessness. In preschool children the main symptom may be a troublesome cough at night. The diagnosis is supported by a history of a triggering factor or of a personal or family history of atopy.

21 E: Cystic fibrosis

Cystic fibrosis is inherited as an autosomal recessive disease. In Caucasians, the carrier rate is 1 in 25. Most children present with malabsorption and failure to thrive from birth, accompanied by recurrent chest infections. Finger clubbing is a feature of established disease. Other features are sinusitis, nasal polyps and rectal prolapse. Older children and adolescents may have diabetes mellitus, cirrhosis or pneumothorax, and boys may be sterile.

Theme: **Abdominal pain**

22 F: Infantile colic

Infantile colic is common in the first few months of life. Paroxysmal uncontrollable crying with drawing up of the knees, takes place several times a day, particularly in the evening. The condition resolves by 4 months of age. Symptomatic advice is helpful.

23 I: Mesenteric adenitis

The associated pain usually resolves within 24–48 hours. It is less severe than appendicitis and tenderness in right iliac fossa is variable. It is accompanied by an upper respiratory tract infection (URTI) and cervical lymphadenopathy.

24   G: Intussusception

Intussusception occurs between 2 months and 2 years of age. It is caused by invagination of the proximal bowel into the distal segment. No underlying intestinal cause is found. A viral illness causing enlargement of Peyer's patches may cause the lead point. Presenting features are a severe, paroxysmal colicky pain and pallor – the child becomes pale, especially around the mouth, and draws the legs up during episodes of pain. A sausage-shaped mass is often palpable in the abdomen. Passage of a stool comprising bloodstained mucus, abdominal distension and shock should be treated with immediate resuscitation and reduction.

25   B: Acute appendicitis

This is the commonest cause of abdominal pain in childhood requiring surgical intervention. Common symptoms are anorexia, vomiting and abdominal pain that is initially central but then localises to the right iliac fossa. Signs are a flushed face with bad breath, fever, tenderness and guarding at McBurney's point. Perforation is common in children as the omentum is less developed and fails to surround the appendix.

26   A: Abdominal migraine

Abdominal pain usually accompanies cranial migraine, but in children the abdominal pain may be the predominant feature. The pain is usually midline, paroxysmal or stereotypic, with facial pallor. Usually, there is a personal or family history of migraine. Pizotifen is a helpful prophylactic agent in children with frequent symptoms.

27   H: Irritable bowel syndrome

This syndrome is associated with altered gastrointestinal motility. There is a positive family history and it is associated with anxiety and stress. It is uncommon in children. Symptoms are bloating, a mucous stool, a feeling of incomplete defecation, constipation alternating with a loose stool, and the relief of pain by defecation.

Theme: Diarrhoea

28 A: Coeliac disease

Coeliac disease is an enteropathy in which gluten provokes a damaging immunological response in the proximal small intestinal mucosa. It commonly presents in the first 2 years of life following the introduction of gluten in cereals. General irritability, abnormal stools, abdominal distension and wasting of the buttocks are common symptoms. In late childhood, children present with anaemia, growth failure and non-gastrointestinal symptoms. Diagnosis is by jejunal biopsy which reveals a flat mucosa (resolves on gluten withdrawal). Anti-endomyseal antibody is useful for screening.

29 D: Toddler's diarrhoea

Toddler's diarrhoea is the commonest cause of persistent loose stools in preschool children. The stool may sometimes be well formed, sometimes explosive and loose. The presence of undigested vegetable in the stool gives it the alternative name of 'peas and carrot syndrome'. The child is usually well and thriving, with no precipitating dietary factor. The condition usually settles by time the child is 5 years old. Usually no treatment is required. Occasionally, loperamide is given (cautiously).

30 B: Crohn's disease

Crohn's disease is a chronic inflammatory disease affecting any part of the GI tract from mouth to anus, but commonly affecting the distal ileum and proximal colon. The affected intestine is thickened, with histology showing non-caseating epithelial-cell granulomas. Common features are diarrhoea, abdominal pain, growth failure and pubertal delay. Oral and perianal ulcers, anal fistulas, skin tags and fissures are common. Other features are arthritis, uveitis and erythema nodosum. Treatment involves suppression of inflammation by steroids or the use of an elemental diet for a period of 6 weeks. In cases of recurrence, azathioprine maintains remission. Complications such as fissure, fistula, obstruction and growth failure require surgery.

31 C: Milk intolerance

This is common in infants with IgA deficiency and a family history of atopy. It usually manifests as diarrhoea, vomiting,

failure to thrive, migraine and eczema, and occasionally with
urticaria, stridor and shock. Jejunal biopsy will show a patchy
enteropathy with prominent eosinophils in the lamina propria.
Most children outgrow their intolerance by 2 years of age.
Avoidance of the offending antigen leads to resolution of
symptoms. Soya milk is often given but 30% of children are
intolerant to soya and hydrolysate-based formula is preferred.

Theme: Painful limbs in children

32   I: Transient synovitis

Transient synovitis is the most common cause of acute hip pain
in children between 2 and 12 years of age. Presentation is with a
sudden-onset pain in the hip or a limp. There is no pain at rest.
Pain may cause a reduced range of movements, particularly
external rotation, and may be referred to the knee. The child may
be febrile but does not appear ill. Neutrophils and acute-phase
reactants are normal or slightly raised. Blood cultures are
negative. Although joint X-rays are normal, a small joint effusion
may be demonstrated on ultrasound. Management is bedrest and
skin traction. It usually improves in a few days.

33   E: Osgood–Schlatter disease

Osgood–Schlatter disease is a syndrome of overuse, commonly
occurring in physically active boys around puberty. It is caused by
the detachment of a fragment of cartilage from the tibial
tuberosity, over which there is localised tenderness and swelling.
Most cases resolve by reducing physical activity. Sometimes
immobilisation and, albeit rarely, excision of the ossicle is
required.

34   H: Slipped femoral epiphysis

There is displacement of the epiphysis of the femoral head
posteroinferiorly. It is common in obese boys between the ages of
5 and 15 years. Presentation is with pain in a hip that may refer to
the knee. Abduction and internal rotation are restricted. Onset

may be acute after a minor trauma. Diagnosis is by X-ray. Management is surgical, usually with pin fixation *in situ*.

35   G: Septic arthritis

Children with septic arthritis have a high fever and look unwell; there is pain at rest or minimal movement of the hip. Neutrophils and acute-phase reactants are markedly raised. The joint should be aspirated under ultrasound guidance if there is a suspicion of septic arthritis. Management of septic arthritis is as follows:

- prolonged course of antibiotics, iv initially then orally
- surgical drainage if delayed resolution or if the sepsis is deep seated (in the hip)
- immobilisation of the affected joint.

36   D: Non-accidental injury

Non-accidental injury is suspected in this case, as a 4-week-old child is incapable of rolling off the bed. In all cases of suspected non-accidental injury (NAI) the policy of the local Child Protection Committee should be followed. A full history and clinical examination should be performed. It should be performed sensitively, without accusing parents. Photographs of the injury should be taken with parental consent. If abuse is suspected the child needs protection from further harm. Hospital admission should be considered for investigation and multidisciplinary team assessment. If parents do not give consent, legal enforcement may be needed. If medical treatment is not needed but there is concern regarding safety of the child, placement of the child may be found in a foster home. Assessment by social workers and health professionals will be needed. A child protection conference will be arranged according to local policy. The conference members will include: social worker, health visitor, paediatrician, GP, teacher, police lawyer. Parents may attend part or all of the conference. The conference will decide the following:

- whether the child will be on the child protection register
- whether there will be an application to the court to protect the child
- follow-up of the child's care.

If the child is put on the child protection register the social services will produce a care plan.

Theme: **Investigations for failure to thrive**

37   C: Chest X-ray and sweat test

Cystic fibrosis is the commonest cause of suppurative lung disease in Caucasians. It is an autosomal recessive disease. Carrier rate is 1 in 25 and incidence is 1 in 2500. A gene located on chromosome 7 codes for a protein called 'cystic fibrosis transmembrane regulator' (CFTR) which is defective in this condition. This results in abnormal ion transport across epithelial cells of exocrine glands of the respiratory system and the pancreas, resulting in increased viscosity of the secretions. As a result the sweat glands produce sweat with an excessive concentration of sodium and chloride (80–125 mmol/l); this forms the basis of the diagnostic test (the sweat test for cystic fibrosis). The increased viscosity of the secretion of the respiratory system leads to blocking of the small airways by viscid mucus, leading to chronic infection and subsequent damage to bronchial walls, in turn leading to bronchiectasis and lung abcess. A chest X-ray is thus performed when cystic fibrosis is suspected.

38   J: Stool microscopy and culture

In a case of intestinal infection stool microscopy and culture helps in identifying the offending agent and decide on management.

39   D: Chromosomal analysis

Turner's syndrome (45,X) has an incidence of 1 in 2500 live-born females. In 50% of girls there are 45 chromosomes with only one X chromosome. The others have a deletion of the short arm of one X chromosome or an isochrome which has two long arms and no short arm or another structural defect of one of the chromosomes. The condition is identified by performing a chromosomal analysis. The clinical features are:
- lymphoedema of the hands and feet in neonates
- webbing of the neck
- short stature
- wide carrying angle and widely spaced nipples
- congenital heart defects (commonly coarctation of the aorta)
- ovarian dysgenesis.

40   B: Anti-endomysial and antigliadin antibodies
Coeliac disease is an enteropathy caused by the gliadin part of gluten which causes immunological damage to the mucosa of the proximal small intestine. The mucosa becomes flat due to loss of the villous tip. Children usually present with failure to thrive after the introduction of cereals to their diet. Children present with irritability, abnormal stool, wasting of buttocks, distended abdomen, anaemia and growth failure. Anti-endomysial antibody and antigliadin antibody tests are useful in screening for this condition but definitive diagnosis is made by jejunal biopsy, which reveals a flat mucosa. This resolves on withdrawl of gluten from the diet.

41   F: Ferritin
In mild iron deficiency the haemoglobin, MCV and MCH may remain normal. As the deficiency progresses MCV and MCH fall and anaemia develops. If iron deficiency is suspected the ferritin level and other indicators of iron stores should be measured.

42   A: Acute-phase reactant
Crohn's disease is a chronic inflammatory disease affecting any part of the gastrointestinal tract from the mouth to the anus, most commonly affecting the distal ileum and proximal colon. The affected loops of bowel are thickened and develop adhesions. Fissures, fistulas and anal tags are common. It may present with abdominal pain, diarrhoea, growth failure, intermittent fever, arthritis, uveitis and erythema nodosum.

Acute-phase reactants (C-reactive protein and ESR) are usually raised and are used to monitor the severity of the disease. Diagnosis is by barium follow-through or colonoscopy, which shows characteristic features such as narrowing, fissuring, mucosal irregularity, and mural thickening of the bowel. Histology of the biopsy shows non-caseating epithelial cell granulomata.

43   K: Thyroid function tests
In hypothyroidism the thyroid function tests show elevated levels of TSH and reduced levels of T3 and T4.

Theme: Respiratory distress in the newborn

44 B: Meconium aspiration

Meconium aspiration affects 25% of deliveries by 42 weeks' gestation. It is passed in response to fetal asphyxia. At birth these infants may inhale thick meconium, which should be aspirated immediately after delivery of the head. Asphyxiated babies may aspirate before delivery. Meconium is a lung irritant and causes both mechanical obstruction and chemical pneumonitis. The lungs are over-inflated with patches of consolidation and collapse. Other complications are pneumothorax and pneumomediastinum. Artificial ventilation is often required.

45 D: Pneumonia

Prolonged membrane rupture, chorioamnionitis and a low birth weight predispose to pneumonia. The cause of infection should be investigated in infants with respiratory distress and broad-spectrum antibiotics started immediately **after** samples are taken, but before the results are available.

46 E: Pneumothorax

Pneumothorax occurs spontaneously in 2% of babies. It can occur secondary to meconium aspiration, RDS and complications of ventilation. Tension pneumothorax is treated by introducing a chest drain. In order to prevent pneumothorax, infants are ventilated at the lowest pressure for adequate chest movement and maintenance of blood gases.

47 C: Milk aspiration

Milk aspiration frequently occurs in preterm infants and those with respiratory distress, neurological damage and cleft palate. Cleft lip can be repaired within a week of birth but cleft palate repair is done at 7 months. Some babies with cleft palate can successfully breast-feed; others require special teats and feeding devices. A dental prosthesis may help until surgical repair.

48 H: Transient tachypnoea

Transient tachypnoea is caused by delay in the resorption of lung liquid. It is more common in babies born by Caesarean section. The chest X-ray may show fluid in the horizontal fissure. The condition usually settles within the first day of life.

49   A: Diaphragmatic hernia
Diaphragmatic hernia in the newborn period usually presents with respiratory distress or a failure to respond to resuscitation. The apex beat and heart sounds are displaced to the right side of chest and there is poor air entry in the left. X-rays of the chest and abdomen confirm the diagnosis. On diagnosis of diaphragmatic hernia, suction is applied with a large nasogastric tube to prevent distension of the bowel. Following stabilisation the hernia is repaired.

Theme: **Screening tests**

50   C: Between a child's fourth and fifth birthdays
Orthoptist assessment of vision is done between the fourth and fifth birthdays to check visual acuity.

51   G: Soon after birth
A general physical examination is done at birth and also at the 6–8-week check-up, with emphasis on the following:
- eyes – check red reflex: absence of the red reflex requires urgent referral to an ophthalmologist
- heart – murmur may need to be investigated for congenital heart defects; infants are referred for USS of heart and to a cardiologist
- hips – checked to rule out congenital dislocation; in case of doubt infants are referred for USS.

52   D: Day 5–6 of life
Blood spot test is done on day 5–6 to identify phenylketonuria and hypothyroidism as early intervention in these conditions leads to a good prognosis and infants whose test is positive are referred to a paediatrician

53   E: In primary school

54   A: At 8 months of age
The infant distraction test is done at 8 months for screening infant hearing. This test relies on the baby locating and turning the ear towards sound. High- and low-frequency sounds are produced outside the child's visual field. This test is unreliable if not carried out by properly trained staff and it is going to be phased out and the automated hearing screen will be done within 1 week to screen infant hearing.

55   H: Within the first week of life
An earpiece is inserted into the ear canal and produces a sound which evokes an echo or emission from the ear if cochlear function is normal.

Theme: **Teratogenic drugs**

56   H: Tetracycline
Tetracycline is deposited in teeth and in growing bone by binding to calcium, and can cause dental staining and growth defects and altered bone growth. Tetracyclines are contraindicated in pregnant or breast-feeding women and in children under 12 years.

57   B: Diethylstilbestrol
Diethylstilbestrol, when given in large doses to pregnant women in the first trimester, has been associated with clear-cell adenocarcinoma of the vagina, an increased risk of infertility and urogenital abnormalities in their daughters, and with hypospadias in their sons.

58   J: Warfarin
Warfarin crosses the placenta and if taken during the first trimester of pregnancy can cause a hypoplastic nasal bridge and chondrodysplasia. During the third trimester warfarin leads to an increased risk of placental or fetal haemorrhage.

59   E: Phenytoin
This anti-epileptic drug is associated with an increased risk of neural tube defects, cleft lip and cleft palate. Pregnant women taking phenytoin should be carefully monitored and should take folic acid supplements.

60 I: Thalidomide

Thalidomide used in the 1950s to treat morning sickness in pregnant women caused disruption and cessation of limb formation in the fetus and the drug was banned in the early 1960s. In the late 1990s it was re-introduced for the treatment of erythema nodosum leprosum in leprosy and in the management of some patients with AIDS/HIV and myeloma. The mechanism of phocomelia is still unknown and there are strict guidelines governing the use of thalidomide in women of childbearing age.

NB. In addition to other textbooks on the subject, refer to the latest edition of the BNF *and read the section on 'Drugs in pregnancy'.*

Paediatric SBAs

1 A 2-month-old baby was brought to the clinic having stopped feeding and with an intermittent high fever. Urine examination shows > 100 white cells/ml and > 10^5 *Escherichia coli*/ml.

What would the SINGLE most appropriate plan of management be?

A   Immediate USS and DMSA scan
B   Initial USS followed by a DMSA scan 3 months later
C   Treat with a 5-day course of trimethoprim with no follow-up
D   Treat with antibiotics followed by a repeat urine culture to check infection
E   Treat with antibiotics, arrange prompt USS, continue prophylactic antibiotics until a DMSA scan and MCUG are done   ☐

2 A 3-year-old child presents with a 3-month history of recurrent episodes of cough and wheeze. The cough is worse at night. Chest examination is normal between episodes of wheeze, but there is prolonged expiratory wheeze during an episode.

What is the SINGLE most appropriate management?

A   Arrange chest X-ray   D   Trial of antihistaminics
B   FBC   E   Trial of bronchodilators
C   Treat with a course of antibiotics   ☐

3 A 5-year-old girl presents at A&E with a severe sore throat, drooling of saliva, high temperature and difficulty in breathing.

What is the SINGLE most appropriate management option?

A   Call the ENT surgeon/senior anaesthetist to secure her airway
B   Lie the child down and examine her throat with a spatula
C   Perform a lateral neck X-ray
D   Prescribe a course of antibiotics and discharge the child
E   Try to intubate the child immediately   ☐

4 A full-term baby appeared jaundiced on day 6. He received a vitamin K injection soon after birth and has been breast-fed from birth. At the age of 4 weeks he presents with poor feeding, vomiting and bruising over his forehead. His urine is dark and his stool is intermittently pale. Investigations show: Hb 8.2 g/dl; platelets 470×10^9/l; prothrombin time grossly prolonged; bilirubin 187 µmol/l, 80% conjugated.

What is the SINGLE most likely diagnosis?

A   Biliary atresia
B   Breast-milk jaundice
C   Crigler–Najjar syndrome

D   G6PD deficiency
E   Hypothyroidism

5 At the postnatal baby check you find that a baby has an asymmetrical skin fold around its hips.

What SINGLE test would you arrange to best confirm the diagnosis?

A   Barlow's test
B   MRI ✓
C   Ortolani's manoeuvre

D   USS ✓
E   X-ray hips

6 An 8-year-old boy complains of aches and pains following exercise; he also says he has difficulty chewing and swallowing. On examination there is a violaceous hue to his eyelids with periorbital oedema.

What is the SINGLE most likely diagnosis?

A   Dermatomyositis
B   Duchenne's muscular dystrophy
C   Fascioscapulohumeral dystrophy

D   Myotonia dystrophica
E   SLE

tx: steroids

7 A 5-year-old child is brought by his parents to see you. They are worried that he wets his bed every night. A urine culture is normal and the urine is negative for glucose and protein.

What would be the SINGLE best management for this child?

A   Desmopressin nasal spray *after 7 ylo*
B   Oral imipramine
C   Prophylactic antibiotics
D   Reassure the parents that it will settle with time
E   Referral to specialist for USS and MCUG   ☐

8 A 5-year-old child complains of difficulty in hearing. He has had several fractures following minor falls. On examination his legs appear short and deformed and his sclera appears blue.

What is the SINGLE most likely diagnosis?

A   Achondroplasia   D   Osteogenesis imperfecta
B   Cleidocranial dystosis   E   Osteopetrosis
C   Marfan's syndrome   ☐

9

What SINGLE condition would be most likely to lead to a suspicion of non-accidental injury?

A   Blue discoloration on the back of a child
B   Mid-clavicular fracture in a 10-day-old child
C   Multiple bruises of various age on the shin of a 5-year-old boy
D   Torn frenulum in a 4-month-old baby
E   Widespread petechial rash in a 2-year-old child   ☐

10 A 4-week-old infant presents with projectile vomiting after feeds. The baby is constantly hungry.

What is the single best management for this condition?

A   Billroth-I operation
B   Negus' hydrostatic bag
C   Positioning in the 30° head-up prone position after feeds
D   Pyloromyotomy
E   Thickening of feeds   ☐

11 Tom, the second child of healthy parents, was born at term by emergency Caesarean section for fetal distress. The pregnancy had been uneventful and the antenatal USS detected no abnormalities. Investigation, because of respiratory distress and cardiac murmur, reveals an interrupted aortic arch and ventricular septal defect that requires surgical correction in the neonatal period. On examination there are minor dysmorphic features, including a short filtrum and thin upper lip and prominent ears.

Which SINGLE statement best fits this scenario?

A   Hypercalcaemia is a constant association of the disease
B   There is no increased risk in subsequent pregnancies
C   There is a deletion on the long arm of chromosome 2
D   Mental retardation is a constant feature for children who survive until adulthood
E   Cytogenetic analysis by fluorescent *in situ* hybridisation is used to detect the condition   FISH

12 A 2-day-old neonate was cyanosed. Umbilical artery blood sampling showed a $p(O_2)$ of 2 kPa. Auscultation of the chest revealed a pulmonary stenosis murmur. Chest X-ray showed a narrow upper mediastinum with an egg-on-side appearance of the cardiac shadow. Balloon atrial septostomy has been performed as a life-saving procedure.

What is the SINGLE most likely diagnosis?

A   Hypoplastic left heart syndrome
B   Interruption of the aortic arch
C   Patent ductus arteriosus
D   Tetralogy of Fallot   boot - shaped
E   Transposition of the great arteries

ↆ Na ↑K

13 A 2-week-old neonate presented with vomiting and weight loss, floppiness and circulatory collapse. Blood testing showed low sodium and high potassium levels. There was a metabolic acidosis and the baby was found to be hypoglycaemic. The paediatrician noticed that the penis was enlarged and the scrotum pigmented. The child was treated with a glucocorticoid and mineralocorticoid.

What is the SINGLE most likely diagnosis?

A   Addisonian crisis

B   Congenital adrenal hyperplasia

C   Conn's syndrome

D   Cushing's syndrome

E   Thyrotoxic crisis

☐

14 A 2-year-old girl was taken to see her GP as her mother had noticed that she had developed a slight squint in her left eye. On examination, the red reflex is absent.   *Retinoblastoma   ch 13*

Which ONE of the following statements best describes this child's condition?

A   It has a very high mortality rate

B   Most cases present after the age of 3 years

C   The gene associated with this condition is located on chromosome 16

D   The pattern of inheritance is recessive

E   There is a significant risk of secondary malignancy in the survivors

sarcoma

☐

15 A baby born at 33 weeks' gestation develops sudden abdominal distension and a purpuric rash and passes blood and mucus per rectum during his first week of life in the SCBU (Special Care Baby Unit).

Which is the SINGLE most likely diagnosis?

A   Gastroschisis

B   Haemolytic-uraemic syndrome

C   Haemorrhagic disease of the newborn

D   Hirschsprung's disease

E   Necrotising enterocolitis

Paediatric SBAs – Answers

1 E: Treat with antibiotics, arrange prompt USS, continue prophylactic antibiotics until a DMSA scan and MCUG are done

The protocol for investigation of a first UTI is as follows:

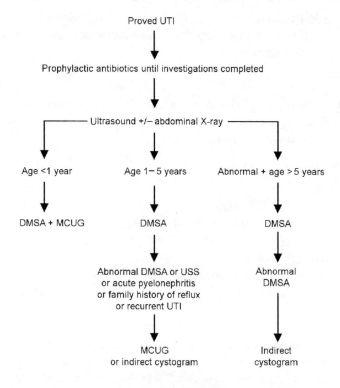

An MCUG (micturating cystourethrogram) should not be performed acutely, as transient reflux may occur following a bladder infection and micturating cystourethrography (MCU) also risks introducing infection. Therefore an MCU should be done a few weeks after a UTI and always under antibiotic cover. A [$^{99}Tc^{m}$]DMSA (technetium 99m-labelled dimercaptosuccinic acid) scan shows areas of renal parenchymal damage and should be deferred for about 3 months after a UTI to avoid missing a newly developed scar, and because false-positives result due to transient reflux or inflammation.

2   E: Trial of bronchodilators

Usually, the diagnosis of asthma is clear from the history and examination, and investigation is not needed. Although a chest X-ray will often show hyperinflation, it will rarely influence management (but a CXR is helpful for excluding congenital anomalies). Children over the age of 5 years can use a peak-flow meter.

3   A: Call the ENT surgeon/senior anaesthetist to secure her airway

This is a clinical picture of acute epiglottitis. Trying to examine the child or trying to intubate, if you are not very experienced, may precipitate airway obstruction. The most appropriate management would be to ask for help from an experienced ENT surgeon or senior anaesthetist.

4   A: Biliary atresia

All these conditions present with prolonged jaundice. Conjugated bilirubinaemia is found in biliary atresia. Neonatal conjugated hyperbilirubinaemia is evaluated by screening for infections, genetic disorders (eg α_1-antitrypsin deficiency, galactosaemia, cystic fibrosis) and metabolic conditions (eg tyrosinaemia):

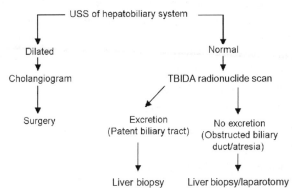

NB. With TBIDA (99m-labelled trimethylbromoiminodiacetic acid) radionuclide scanning, the isotope is picked up by the liver cells and excreted into the bowel. However, in the case of extrahepatic biliary obstruction or biliary atresia or in cases of severe extrahepatic

cholestasis, the isotope is not excreted into the bowel.

5 D: USS

You could confirm the diagnosis of congenital dysplasia of the hip (CDH) with USS or MRI, or with an arthrogram. However, USS is used to rule out CDH, whereas Barlow's and Ortolani's tests are used to screen for this condition. As an X-ray doesn't show ossification centres in neonates, it is not helpful before the age of 6 weeks.

6 A: Dermatomyositis

This is a more benign condition in children than it is in adults. There is symmetrical ascending weakness and the trunk muscles and flexors of the neck are typically involved. Bulbar muscle involvement causes problems with chewing and swallowing. A violaceous hue to the upper eyelid and oedema of the eyelids are classic features of the condition. The ESR (erythrocyte sedimentation rate) and creatinine kinase level may be normal or raised. Muscle biopsy reveals an inflammatory cell infiltrate. Steroids are the treatment of choice; azathioprine or ciclosporin may be tried if the response is poor. Around 50% of affected children recover.

7 D: Reassure the parents that it will settle with time

Some 15% of children suffer from enuresis at the age of 5 years: 5% of 10-year-olds and 1% of 15-year-olds still wet the bed. The boy:girl ratio is 2:1. Treatment is not undertaken until a child is 6 years of age. In this case, both the child and parents should be given an explanation and reassurance. Star charts and an enuresis alarm are effective in motivated children. Desmopressin, either in the form of tablets or a spray, is prescribed for children over 7 years of age. Imipramine is avoided due to its side-effects and the risk of overdose.

8 D: Osteogenesis imperfecta

There are two types of osteogenesis imperfecta:
* Type 1 – the more common, has an autosomal dominant pattern of inheritance. Frequent fractures occur during childhood. Common features are bow-legs and blue discoloration of the sclera. Affected children may develop hearing loss. The prognosis is variable. Any fracture requires splinting to reduce deformity.

- Type 2 – more lethal, with multiple fractures already present before birth. Many babies are stillborn. Inheritance may be autosomal dominant, or it may be the result of a new mutation.

9   D: Torn frenulum in a 4-month-old baby

A mid-clavicular fracture in a 10-day-old baby is most likely to be the result of a difficult delivery and a history of the mode of birth should be taken. Although a facial petechial rash may be a sign of smothering, it could be due to cough, as in whooping cough. A generalised petechial rash should raise the suspicion of idiopathic thrombocytopenic purpura or meningococcal septicaemia. A blue discoloration on the back of an infant is Mongolian blue spot. It is a harmless congenital blue marking on the buttock or sacrum and is commonly mistaken for abuse. Bruises of different ages in a 5-year-old child is a normal finding, but would be suspicious if the child was less than 7 months of age.

Common signs of a suspicious non-accidental injury are bite marks, a torn frenulum from forced bottle-feeding, ligature marks, and burns and scalds.

10   D: Pyloromyotomy

The incidence of pyloric stenosis is 4 per 1000 births, boys being affected more than girls in the ratio of 4:1. Some 15% of affected infants have a family history. Vomiting is projectile and occurs after feeds, but is not bile-stained as the obstruction is so high. Examination will reveal an olive-shaped mass in the upper abdomen during test feeds. USS is the investigation of choice. Treatment is surgical, by Ramstedt's pylorotomy.

11   E: Cytogenetic analysis by fluorescent *in situ* hybridisation (FISH) is used to detect the condition

This condition arises as the result of a developmental defect of derivatives of the third and fourth pharyngeal pouches. It is almost always associated with agenesis or hypoplasia of the thymus and parathyroid gland, characteristic facies with down-slanting palpebral fissures and ocular and nasal anomalies, hypocalcaemia, cardiovascular anomalies, immunodeficiency and other variable abnormalities. Patients who survive infancy are usually mentally retarded. The DiGeorge syndrome is considered by some researchers to be a developmental field defect consisting of several causally distinct disorders, rather than a distinct syndromic entity. Conditions associated with the development of the DiGeorge syndrome include diabetic embryopathy, fetal alcohol syndrome and the Zellweger syndrome. Major features of this syndrome have been designated by the Newcastle-upon-Tyne Group as 'CATCH 22' (Cardiac, Abnormal facies, Thymic hypoplasia, Cleft palate and Hypocalcaemia), the number 22 indicating deletion on the long arm of chromosome 22 (22q11). There is an increased risk of this condition in subsequent pregnancies.

12　E: Transposition of the great arteries

Affected children usually present in the first day or two of life, with the spontaneous closure of the ductus arteriosus leading to a marked reduction in the mixing of desaturated and saturated blood. An ECG is rarely helpful in establishing the diagnosis. Echocardiography is essential to demonstrate the abnormal arterial connection and associated abnormalities. Maintaining the patency of the ductus arteriosus with prostaglandin infusion is mandatory.

13　B: Congenital adrenal hyperplasia

Congenital adrenal hyperplasia has an incidence of 1 in 5000. It has an autosomal recessive pattern of inheritance and is common in the offspring of consanguineous marriages. Some 90% of cases are due to deficiency of the enzyme 21-hydroxylase, which is needed for cortisol synthesis. In 80% of cases there is failure of aldosterone production. Affected females require corrective surgery of the external genitalia.

14　E: There is a significant risk of secondary malignancy in the survivors

Retinoblastoma accounts for about 5% of cases of severe visual impairment in children. The suspected gene is located on chromosome 13 and the mode of inheritance is dominant. Children from families that suffer from the hereditary form should undergo regular screening. The commonest presentation is with a white pupillary reflex or a squint. Treatment is with chemotherapy to shrink the tumour, followed by laser therapy to the retina to preserve vision. Although most patients are cured, many suffer from impaired vision. There is a significant risk of secondary malignancy in survivors, especially of sarcoma.

15   E: Necrotising enterocolitis

Necrotising enterocolitis is common in preterm babies. It typically affects babies in SCBU at the end of the first week of life. Clinical features vary from the passage of a little blood and mucus per rectum in mild cases to perforation, shock, disseminated intravascular coagulation (DIC) and sloughing of the rectal mucosa in severe cases. Investigations performed are stool culture and supine and erect abdominal X-rays, which show oedematous loops of bowel with intramural gas. Treatment for mild cases includes barrier nursing and stopping oral feeding. In severe cases, intravenous antibiotics (metronidazole + penicillin + netilmicin) should be given, blood should be cross-matched and the baby referred to a surgeon for laparotomy.

Psychiatry

Chapter contributed by
Dr Rahul Bhattacharya MBBS DPM

Psychiatry EMQs

Theme: **Questionnaires**

Options

A AUDIT *Alc. use disorder ident. tst*
B BDI *Beck's dep. inventory*
C CAGE
D Edinburgh PND scale
E GHQ *gen health questionnaire*
F MMSE
G PANSS *(+)+(−) synd scale*
H PSE *present state exam*
I WAIS *16–89 y/o*
J WAIS-III *5–15 y/o*

Instructions

For each of the patients described below choose the SINGLE most appropriate questionnaire from the list of options above. Each option may be used once, more than once or not at all.

1 A 32-year-old patient attends your surgery and you want to check for alcohol problems. ☐

2 A 32-year-old woman recently gave birth to her first child and you want to screen for postnatal depression. ☐

3 A 78-year-old woman attends the memory clinic for review of donepezil. ☐

4 You want to carry out a survey of your local population to screen for general psychiatric morbidity. ☐

5 A 7-year-old boy attends your surgery who you suspect has some learning difficulties. ☐

Theme: **Diagnosis of personality**

Options

A   Antisocial personality traits
B   Borderline personality traits
C   Extroverted personality
D   Introverted personality
E   Paranoid personality traits
F   Schizoid personality traits
G   Schizotypal personality traits
H   Type A personality
I   Type B personality
J   Type C personality

Instructions

For each of the patients described below choose the SINGLE most appropriate personality diagnosis from the list of options above. Each option may be used once, more than once or not at all.

6   A 49-year-old unmarried man, who has worked as a cleaner in a Scottish skiing resort for the past 29 years, has recently found it difficult to cope with his work. His mother died 3 months ago. He has not been in touch with his family and has few friends. This man has refused an offer by his same employers to work as a cleaning supervisor at a hotel in Glasgow.

7   A 20-year-old medical student is severely upset by her grades in year 2 of medical school, even though her parents say her grades are 'reasonably good'. She has had problems with her friends on a couple of occasions in the past.

8   A 17-year-old boy has been permanently excluded from his course after he poured some acid on one of his friends. He finds this 'funny' and feels the college is over-reacting. He is known to tease his cat and experiment with illicit drugs.

9   A 19-year-old man doing a part-time IT course is finding it extremely difficult to approach a woman on the same course, even though she appears to be friendly. He has few friends and enjoys listening to music.

10   A 22-year-old girl is presently in her third relationship, which she describes as volatile. She took an overdose after a recent fall. Her boyfriend has observed mood fluctuations that are difficult to deal with, and has observed several scars of possible self-inflicted injuries.

Theme: **Management in substance misuse**

Options

A	Acamprosate	G	Methadone
B	Buprenorphine	H	Naloxone
C	Bupropion	I	Naltrexone
D	Buspirone	J	Urinalysis for substance
E	Diazepam		identification and observation
F	Lofexidine		of withdrawal symptoms

Instructions

For each of the patients described below choose the SINGLE most appropriate treatment from the list of options above. Each option may be used once, more than once or not at all.

11 A 45-year-old man, having been involved in a road traffic accident, was motivated to abstain from alcohol. He has successfully undergone detoxification but is having problems dealing with craving.

12 A 24-year-old man has presented to A&E demanding methadone 40 mg as he says he is withdrawing from his heroin addiction. He has no previous drug records but claims he takes 20 mg intravenous heroin a day.

13 A 37-year-old teacher, with no obvious findings on medical check-up, is requesting help to give up cigarette smoking.

14 A 69-year-old woman has been on temazepam 20 mg as night-time sedation for the past 20 years. Recently, she watched a TV programme reporting that these tablets are addictive, but says she would not like to come off them.

15 A 25-year-old heroin addict is undergoing inpatient detoxification, aiming for abstinence. What medication would you use to deal with her opioid withdrawal?

Theme: **Memory difficulties**

Options

A	Anterograde amnesia	F	False-memory syndrome
B	Confabulation	G	Patchy amnesia
C	Dissociative amnesia	H	Post-traumatic amnesia
D	Dissociative fugue	I	Retrograde amnesia
E	*En bloc* amnesia	J	Transient global amnesia

Instructions

For each of the patients described below choose the SINGLE most appropriate diagnosis from the list of options above. Each option may be used once, more than once or not at all.

16 A 36-year-old man has been identified by his sister. For the past 3 days he has reportedly been missing from Birmingham after he broke up with his girlfriend. He has no recollection of anything, including who he is. ☐

17 A 24-year-old man in ITU cannot remember the events leading up to his RTA, following which he was admitted, 2 weeks ago. He only remembers waking up in his ITU bed yesterday. ☐

18 A 23-year-old woman wakes up at her friend's place on Sunday afternoon after an alcoholic binge on Saturday night. She cannot remember anything after the first few hours at the party. ☐

19 A 54-year-old man, recovering from Korsakoff's psychosis in a rehabilitation ward, mentions how he was visiting the pyramids by camel this morning. ☐

20 A 63-year-old man recovered completely the day after he failed to remember anything the day before. However, he always knew who he was. ☐

Theme: **Dementia and organic psychiatry**

Options

A	Alzheimer's disease	F	Lewy body dementia
B	Binswanger's disease	G	Parkinson's dementia
C	Delirium	H	Pick's disease
D	Frontotemporal dementia	I	Wilson's disease
E	Huntington's disease		

Instructions

For each of the patients described below choose the SINGLE most appropriate diagnosis from the list of options above. Each option may be used once, more than once or not at all.

21 A 76-year-old patient is recovering from a hip replacement operation in a London hospital. For the past 2 days she has been taking out her fluid line and insisting on going to Ireland. The nurses have noticed that her symptoms are worse in the evening.

22 A 76-year-old man with a history of fluctuating consciousness and visual hallucinations became extremely stiff and had a fall after being given 0.5 mg risperidone to treat his hallucinations.

23 An 80-year-old woman lives alone. She is finding it difficult to remember names. Recently, she had to be collected from the police station after she lost her way back from the supermarket.

24 A 59-year-old man has been seen behaving inappropriately over the last 2 months and has recently exposed himself in public. Recently, he has also been observed to be incontinent.

25 A 37-year-old man has been seen behaving oddly, with abnormal movements and memory problems. On investigation, his liver functions were found to be compromised.

Theme: **Risk assessment as a psychiatric SHO**

Options

A   Admit
B   Advise to inform the police
C   Ask to come to A&E
D   Assess using a risk assessment tool
E   Detain under the emergency Mental Health Act for 72 hours
F   Offer haloperidol im
G   Offer im lorazepam and haloperidol
H   Offer oral haloperidol and lorazepam
I   Request for Mental Health Act assessment
J   Review when medically fit and awake
K   Seclusion

Instructions

For each of the patients described below choose the SINGLE most appropriate management from the list of options above. Each option may be used once, more than once or not at all.

26 A 30-year-old man is referred to you by the casualty officer. The patient was brought in having taken an overdose of 39 amitriptyline tablets. He is drowsy and has cardiac arrhythmia. ☐

27 A 49-year-old patient in your local secure unit (forensic psychiatric ward) has assaulted a member of staff and remains agitated. Verbal de-escalation has not been effective. He has a history of neuroleptic malignant syndrome. The member of staff is not seriously injured and does not want to press charges. ☐

28 An anxious mother has called the ward to seek help. Her 23-year-old son, a known heroin and cocaine addict, is smashing up the house and demanding money. ☐

29 A 36-year-old woman, who was informally admitted to the acute psychiatric ward last week following a serious overdose, is demanding to be discharged over the weekend. She is ambivalent about suicidal intent and her family is not contactable. ☐

30 A 27-year-old man with history of schizophrenia is refusing all
contact with the psychiatric team. His mother is concerned that
he is neither eating nor sleeping well and his flat is in an
unhygienic state.   ☐

Theme: **Investigations in psychiatry**

Options

A	Alkaline phosphatase (blood)	G	Glucose (blood)
B	Carbohydrate-depleted transferrin	H	Mid-stream urine for UTI
		I	MRI
C	Creatinine phosphokinase (blood)	J	Prolactin level (blood)
		K	RBC transketolase
D	CT scan	L	Thyroid profile (blood)
E	EEG	M	Urea and creatinine (blood)
F	GGT	N	Urinalysis for drugs

Instructions

For each of the patients described below choose the SINGLE most appropriate investigation from the list of options above. Each option may be used once, more than once or not at all.

31 A 35-year-old, slightly obese, depressed woman has not responded to a trial of fluoxetine and then venlafaxine.

32 A 24-year-old man appears stiff and has a raised temperature after receiving zuclopenthixol and haloperidol following his first admission.

33 You suspect that a 32-year-old woman is suffering from non-epileptiform seizures.

34 An investigation that is relatively specific for delirium tremens.

35 You want to ascertain recent alcohol use in a person with chronic hepatitis.

Theme: **Side-effects of medication**

Options

A	Arrhythmia	G	Neural tube abnormalities
B	Bone marrow suppression	H	Neuroleptic malignant syndrome
C	Cheese reaction	I	Neutropenia
D	Discontinuation syndrome	J	Obesity
E	Hypothyroidism	K	Serotonin syndrome
F	Liver dysfunction		

Instructions

For each of the patients described below choose the SINGLE most appropriate side-effect from the list of options above. Each option may be used once, more than once or not at all.

36 A 34-year-old woman has been taking lithium for the past 4 years.

37 A 27-year-old woman has developed symptoms of irritability, restlessness, sweating, increased muscle tone and myoclonus while her medications are being switched.

38 A 29-year-old woman with bipolar affective disorder is taking semi-sodium valproate for prophylaxis of her illness. This poses a risk if she gets pregnant.

39 A risk one should be aware of in a 62-year-old man on amitriptyline.

40 A side-effect of MAO inhibitors that should be borne in mind.

Theme: **Diagnosis of mental illness**

Options

A	Autism	G	Narcolepsy
B	Bipolar affective disorder	H	Psychotic depression
C	Catalepsy	I	Schizoid personality
D	Childhood schizophrenia	J	Schizophrenia
E	Delirium	K	Wernicke's encephalopathy
F	Delirium tremens		

48 – 72 h

Instructions

For each of the patients described below choose the SINGLE most appropriate diagnosis from the list of options above. Each option may be used once, more than once or not at all.

41 A 36-year-old man who believes his gut is rotting has not been eating for this reason. He also hears voices saying that he is dead.

42 A 21-year-old man recently realised, after weeks of having an uneasy feeling and anxiety, that aliens have set up a special link with him to act as a liaison person for planet Earth.

43 A 7-year-old boy has a peculiar attachment to a chair, has continued nocturnal enuresis, has a vocabulary of seven words and avoids eye contact.

44 An 8-year-old boy reports having briefly seen two men looking at him from beside his bed after he woke up, and for a moment he felt he could not move.

45 A 56-year-old man, admitted to hospital 2 days ago after a road traffic accident, has become increasingly fearful and restless, and is complaining of small people walking along the ceiling. He has a raised pulse rate, fluctuating consciousness and labile blood pressure.

Theme: **Choice of appropriate management**

Options

A	Clomipramine	G	Non-psychopharmacological
B	Dosulepin		management
C	Fluoxetine	H	Olanzapine
D	Imipramine	I	Paroxetine
E	Lithium	J	Pindolol
F	Moclobemide	K	Sertraline

MAOI – A

Instructions

For each of the patients described below choose the SINGLE most appropriate management from the list of options above. Each option may be used once, more than once or not at all.

46 A 15-year-old girl presents to the services for the first time with restrictive eating habits, distorted body image, a target weight of 39 kg and a BMI of 17. ☐

47 A 40-year-old man becomes extremely anxious when attending meetings, and flushes disproportionately when asked to speak. ☐

48 A 15-year-old boy presents with irritability, low mood and self-harming behaviour. ☐

49 A 21-year-old woman presents with severe premenstrual tension that affects her functioning. ☐

50 A 7-year-old boy presenting with nocturnal enuresis is not responding to behavioural management. ☐

Psychiatry EMQs – Answers

Theme: Questionnaires

1 C: CAGE

This is a screening questionnaire devised to identify problematic drinking in an outpatient department or primary care setting. It comprises a four-item questionnaire about: Cutting down drinking; Annoyed by criticism; Guilty about drinking; Eye-opener drink – needing a drink first thing in the morning. Positive answers to two or more questions is indicative of problem drinking.

2 D: Edinburgh PND scale

The Edinburgh Post-Natal Depression Scale is a ten-item self-reporting questionnaire used to screen for postnatal depression.

3 F: MMSE

The Mini-Mental State Examination is a 30-item objective assessment test that can be used to screen for Alzheimer's disease (AD) as well as to monitor prognosis. A score below 26 is usually indicative of mild AD. Recent National Institute for Clinical Excellence (NICE) guidelines recommend the prescription of anti-dementia medication for patients with MMSE scores between 26 and 12.

4 E: GHQ

The General Health Questionnaire is a screening tool devised to identify psychiatric morbidity in a population.

5 J: WAIS-III

The Wechsler Adult Intelligence Scale–III is valid for use with 5–15-year-olds, whereas WAIS is designed for 16–89-year-olds. It is the most commonly used intelligence test, and has a variety of sub-tests that are divided into 'performance' and 'verbal' domains.

NB. The BDI (Beck's Depression Inventory) is a self-reporting questionnaire for depression; there is a similar questionnaire for anxiety – BAI. The acronym AUDIT stands for Alcohol-Use Disorder Identification Test, which was devised by the World Health Organisation and is more sensitive than CAGE. PSE stands for Present State Examination and GHQ for General Health Questionnaire, both are instruments used to identify psychiatric morbidity. PANSS is Positive And Negative Syndrome Scale, used for identifying positive and negative symptoms of schizophrenia.

Theme: Diagnosis of personality

6 F: Schizoid personality trait

This is characterised by aloofness, preference for solitude, lack of interest in sexual activities, indifference to others, lack of close friendship and insensitivity to social norms.

7 H: Type A personality

An alternative classification of personality traits into Types A and B has been suggested based on behavioural responses. Type A is characterised by competitiveness and achievement orientation, urgency, aggressiveness and hostility – it has been associated with an increased risk of high blood pressure and coronary heart disease. Type B is characterised by a laid-back and relaxed attitude. Recently, a Type C personality has been added, which is characterised by reserved behaviour and suppressed emotions. It has been suggested that a Type C personality is associated with an increased risk of cancer.

8 A: Antisocial personality trait

Note that 'antisocial' is an American term (see DSM-4, *Diagnostic and Statistical Manual*, 4th edition) while 'dissocial' is a WHO term (see ICD-10, *International Classification of Diseases*, 10th edition). This category involves features of irresponsible behaviour, lack of concern for others or social norms, low frustration tolerance, superficial relationships and lack of remorse.

9 D: Introverted personality

Eysenck suggested an alternative way of looking at personality, with people lying along an extroversion/introversion spectrum. Introversion would involve quiet, thoughtful, passive, careful and reserved features, whereas an extroverted person would be active, sociable and outgoing.

10 B: Borderline personality trait
This involves features of unstable, intense relationships, with a fear of abandonment. There is impulsivity, and self-harming behaviour, feelings of emptiness and disturbed identity. Transient psychotic experiences and co-morbid mood disturbances are common. Also remember a diagnosis of personality disorder needs to establish that the traits are enduring and were developed during the formative years, ie they can be traced back to adolescence or early adulthood.

Theme: **Management in substance misuse**

11 A: Acamprosate
Naltrexone is an alternative, but it is more popular in the US and is not licensed for this purpose in the UK (see *BNF*).

12 J: Urinalysis for substance identification and observation of withdrawal symptoms
Methadone should never be prescribed without evidence of opioid dependence because of the risk of opioid overdose in a naïve patient.

13 C: Bupropion
Bupropion is a noradrenaline- and dopamine-reuptake inhibitor, which was originally launched in the US as an antidepressant but is now licensed in the UK for smoking cessation purposes (see *BNF*).

14 E: Diazepam
Withdrawal should be slow, by moving the patient to longer-acting benzodiazepines.

15 F: Lofexidine
Lofexidine is similar to clonidine, but is better tolerated. It is licensed in the UK for the purpose described in the question.

Buprenorphine is a partial opioid agonist and deemed to be safer. Theoretically, it should not produce a 'buzz' but, in practice, it is still not used as often as methadone.

Theme: Memory difficulties

16 D: Dissociative fugue
The only amnesia where personal identity is lost is dissociative amnesia. However, if this is accompanied by travelling, then a diagnosis of dissociative fugue should be made.

17 H: Post-traumatic amnesia
Post-traumatic amnesia is defined as the interval between the injury and the return of day-to-day memory.

18 E: *En bloc* amnesia
Alcohol intoxication frequently leads to short-term amnesia or blackouts. It can be 'state-dependent', ie memory returns when the person is next intoxicated; 'fragmentary' when there are islets of memory preserved; or *en bloc*, when there is a clearly demarcated memory loss that is not recovered over time.

19 B: Confabulation
Confabulation is associated with frontal lobe disease or confusional states other than the Korsakoff syndrome. It can range from a spontaneous erroneous outpouring of fantastic memory to fleeting distortions in memory when challenged.

20 J: Transient global amnesia
Transient global amnesia is thought to be a vascular phenomenon where all memory may be disrupted other than personal identity.

NB. The false-memory syndrome is associated with the recovery of repressed memory, often tempered by suggestions and wishes, eg in psychotherapy.

Theme: Dementia and organic psychiatry

21 C: Delirium
This is also called 'acute confusional state', and is often associated

with the phenomenon of 'sundowning' as described in the scenario.

22   F: Lewy body dementia

The classic triad of LBD consists of fluctuating consciousness, visual hallucinations and spontaneous parkinsonism. Patients are very susceptible to extrapyramidal symptoms on relatively small doses of neuroleptics, which can be serious. Lewy bodies are found extensively in the cortex (in Parkinson's disease more around the substantia nigra in the subcortical region). Although cholinesterase (ChE) inhibitors have been found to be effective, they are not yet licensed for this use.

23   A: Alzheimer's disease

Remember the four **A**s of classic dementia: **A**mnesia, **A**gnosia, **A**phasia and **A**praxia.

24   D: Frontotemporal dementia

Pick's disease is a particular and rare variant of frontotemporal dementia but FTD has a relatively earlier age of onset.

25   I: Wilson's disease

Always suspect Huntington's disease or Wilson's disease in dementia of early onset associated with movement disorder; suspect early-onset dementia as well (not associated with movement disorders). Family history and genetic counselling are of great significance in early-onset dementias.

NB. Binswanger's disease is also called 'progressive small-vessel disease' – a subcortical dementia associated with cognitive slowing.

Theme: Risk assessment as a psychiatric SHO

26   J: Review when medically fit and awake

The new NICE (National Institute of Clinical Excellence) guidelines suggest that in every case of attempted self-harm the patient should be offered psychiatric review, but you need to deal with the medical emergency first. Psychiatric assessment is offered once the patient is stable medically. Also, if the patient is confused, his mental state will not be stable and risk assessment cannot be carried out in such circumstances.

27 K: Seclusion

A patient is admitted into a secure/locked unit if the risks are considered high. There are usually local management protocols for handling such 'incidents' of assault, with non-pharmacological methods preferred over pharmacological (ie 'rapid tranquilisation'). The risks of tranquilisation in this patient are particularly high because of his history of neuroleptic malignant syndrome and therefore one would initially attempt to manage him by separating him into a safe and calm room, often with closed-circuit television monitoring, called 'seclusion'. Tranquilisation is usually carried out with a combination of neuroleptics and benzodiazepines.

28 B: Advise to inform the police

This person is in the community and the mother is at risk. The police are the only professionals who have the training to intervene at this point. If the police feel they can manage, then involve Mental Health Act professionals at a later stage. One should always remember about ensuring one's own safety and the safety of other members of the team.

29 E: Detain under the emergency Mental Health Act for 72 hours

There is an obvious risk associated in this case, with a recent serious suicide attempt, and that risk is ongoing in the absence of an after-care plan or support in the community. The emergency detention is usually followed up by a formal Mental Health Act assessment, which is carried out by two doctors and an approved social worker.

30 I: Request for a Mental Health Act assessment

This is an unwell patient with a known serious mental illness and a risk of self-neglect, who is not engaging with his treatment. One would admit him with a view to reducing the risk of self-neglect and in order to alleviate his symptoms.

Theme: **Investigations in psychiatry**

31 L: Thyroid profile
Hypothyroidism should always be ruled out in patients who are depressed.

32 C: Creatinine phosphokinase
Along with a raised white cell count, this is a non-specific marker for the neuroleptic malignant syndrome.

33 J: Prolactin level
This differentiates non-epileptiform seizures and epilepsy, providing the prolactin level is measured within 20 minutes of the seizure. Non-epileptiform seizures are not associated with the increased prolactin level seen in epilepsy. However, interpretation is often difficult in the absence of known baseline levels.

34 K: RBC transketolase
This test is rarely used in practice, and diagnosis is often essentially clinical.

35 B: Carbohydrate-depleted transferrin
This is relatively unaffected in patients with liver damage.

Theme: **Side-effects of medication**

36 E: Hypothyroidism
Lithium can cause thyroid disorders and therefore the *British National Formulary* recommends that thyroid function should be measured every 6–12 months. (Also note that lithium has a narrow therapeutic index and serum lithium levels should be monitored to maintain them at 0.4–1.0 mmol/l. Levels above 1.5 mmol/l are dangerous and are associated with coarse tremors, ataxia, renal impairment and convulsions. Lithium should be withdrawn immediately, and sodium-rich fluid administered to reverse its effects. If levels are over 2 mmol/l, then treatment should be carried out in an intensive care setting.)

37 K: Serotonin syndrome
The symptoms described in the scenario are characteristic of the serotonin syndrome, common when two serotonergic drugs are

simultaneously administered, eg switching antidepressants. The symptoms overlap with those of the neuroleptic malignant syndrome (NMS) and can, albeit rarely, be fatal. (See *BNF*.)

38   G: Neural tube abnormalities
There is an increased risk of neural tube defects in babies born to mothers taking valproate (also occurs with those on carbamazepine or other anti-epileptics). Folic acid supplementation is therefore advised before and during pregnancy to counteract this risk.

39   A: Arrhythmia
ECG monitoring is recommended as arrhythmias are a major risk with amitriptyline therapy, and are also associated with abrupt withdrawal of the medication. Other side-effects include urinary retention, angle-closure glaucoma and postural hypotension. Liver dysfunction should ring a cautionary bell for many medications, including amitriptyline, but is less specific. Liver dysfunction can sometimes occur but hepatic failure is not common.

40   C: Cheese reaction
MAOIs are inhibitors of monoamine oxidase. They inhibit the metabolism of monoamine-containing drugs (eg decongestants and cough preparations) as well as foods rich in tyramine (mature cheese, pickled herring, broad beans, etc). This causes the accumulation of amines and results in a dangerous rise of blood pressure – the 'cheese reaction'. The effects persist for up to 2 weeks after taking an MAOI.

Theme: Diagnosis of mental illness

41   H: Psychotic depression
The symptoms described are typical of nihilistic delusion. Nihilistic delusions are pessimistic delusions, eg one is going to die, or even a part of the body is dead, one has no money or the world is coming to an end. Nihilistic delusions are associated with extremes of depressed mood.

42   J: Schizophrenia

This disorder is very heterogeneous in presentation. Symptoms can be clustered into ones where there is loss of a sense of reality, associated with disorganisation and apathy (the latter are the negative symptoms). The reality distortions involve delusions or faulty beliefs, and hallucinations or faulty perceptions, and together comprise the positive symptoms (a more specific list is included in the classifications of symptoms for diagnosis). The symptom described here is suggestive of what can be considered as bizarre delusion and also hints towards thought-broadcast experience, both of which are included in the diagnostic criteria given in ICD-10 and DSM-4.

43   A: Autism

Autism is a disorder that presents with three clusters of features: difficulties in social relationships, difficulties with language development and ritualistic tendencies. It is often associated with abnormal attachment to inanimate objects and developmental delays. The nocturnal enuresis is suggestive of a generalised developmental delay, as in this case.

44   G: Narcolepsy

The symptoms described in this scenario are of sleep paralysis and hypnopompic hallucinations. Cataplexy – or a sudden loss of muscle tone – is common; catalepsy, on the other hand, is an extrapyramidal sign seen in patients with catatonic schizophrenia.

45   F: Delirium tremens

Delirium tremens (DT) is precipitated within 48–72 hours of abstinence in a chronic heavy drinker, and is common after emergency hospital admission where a background history of alcohol use is often unavailable. Vivid hallucinations, particularly visual hallucinations involving Lilliputian images, are classic. However, tactile or auditory hallucinations are not uncommon. Fearful affect, perceptual misinterpretations and delusions are common. There is disorientation and fluctuating consciousness with autonomic hyperactivity. Delirium is a blanket diagnosis that would cover DT, but it is less specific and therefore not the 'most likely' answer.

Theme: Choice of appropriate management

46 G: Non-psychopharmacological management
The first-line management of anorexia nervosa involves psychological interventions (see NICE guidelines, 2004).

47 I: Paroxetine
The diagnosis here is one of social phobia. Although most selective serotonin-reuptake inhibitors (SSRIs) would be expected to be effective, paroxetine is the drug of choice as it has a licence for use in this condition (see *BNF*).

48 C: Fluoxetine
Following recent reports of increased self-harming behaviour in under-18-year-olds taking paroxetine, the only SSRI that retains its use for antidepressant pharmacotherapy in this age group is fluoxetine.

49 C: Fluoxetine
A 70% reduction in premenstrual irritability and low mood is obtained using fluoxetine and clomipramine, suggesting serotonergic imbalance as a possible contributor.

50 D: Imipramine
Imipramine is licensed for use in cases of nocturnal enuresis, providing anatomical abnormalities have been ruled out. However, medication is usually limited to brief periods to cover for occasions such as going on holiday. Desmopressin is an alternative to imipramine for this purpose.

Psychiatry SBAs

1 A 27-year-old professional man, presently stable on 20 mg fluoxetine treatment for mild depression, is seeking advice about resuming driving his car.

Which SINGLE recommendation by the DVLA applies in this case?

A   A licence is usually refused
B   He can resume driving if there is no other complication
C   He should refrain from driving for 6 months
D   He should refrain from driving for 12 months
E   He should refrain from driving pending a medical report ☐

2

Which SINGLE feature should a screening tool for an easy-to-treat disease possess?

A   Be exhaustive   D   Have high sensitivity
B   Does not need to be reliable   E   Have high specificity
C   Have high internal validity   ☐

3 A 45-year-old man has been referred for rehabilitation following a closed head injury sustained in a road traffic accident.

While assessing him, what SINGLE indication should be remembered as being a poor marker of the severity of the head injury?

A   Anterograde amnesia   *loss of ability to create new memorie*
B   Duration of loss of consciousness
C   Glasgow Coma Scale score following head injury
D   Post-traumatic amnesia
E   Retrograde amnesia   ☐
        └ failure to remember events leading up to an event or injury

4 A 57-year-old woman, who is in an intensive care unit following a myocardial infarction 36 hours ago, has become increasingly confused and is disorientated. She is refusing medication and wanting to go home.

Which is the SINGLE most appropriate course of action in this scenario, considering she is refusing treatment?

A She can be detained under the Mental Health Act to receive treatment
B She can be treated with her best interests in mind ('common law')
C She cannot be treated under any condition
D She should be restrained to provide treatment
E The Trust solicitor should be contacted

5 A 67-year-old man with a long history of suffering from schizophrenia is planning to make his will. You have been asked to assess his capacity to make a valid will.

What SINGLE circumstance precludes him from making a will?

A He does not know the extent of his belongings
B He has no relatives
C He is deluded
D He is detained under the Mental Health Act
E He is refusing medication

6 The parents of a 4-year-old boy report that he wakes and, at times, screams in the middle of the night. However, he goes back to sleep on his own and has no recollection of the events the following day. His father is known to have had similar experiences as a child.

What is the SINGLE most likely diagnosis?

A Childhood depression   D Nightmares
B Ill-formed dreams   E Somnambulism
C Night terrors   *Sleep-walking*

non-REM
familial

7 You have been asked to see a 5-year-old boy by his parents. The boy has mutilated lips, performs head banging and exhibits aggressive behaviour. He also suffers from seizures and abnormal movements. His parents say they are no longer able to cope with the situation.

What SINGLE condition are you most likely to be dealing with here?

A   Down's syndrome   D   Prader–Willi syndrome   *Chr 15*
B   Hurler's syndrome   *Reilly*   E   Tay–Sachs disease   *AR*
C   Lesch–Nyhan syndrome   *bodies*

8 A 15-year-old boy presents with learning disability with autistic features.

What is the single most UNLIKELY possible diagnosis?

A   Asperger's disease   D   Tuberous sclerosis
B   Down's syndrome   E   Turner's syndrome
C   Fragile X syndrome

9 A 23-year-old mother has been observed by the health visitor to be rather weepy 3 days following the delivery of her baby.

What is the SINGLE most likely diagnosis?

A   Depression   D   Puerperal blues   *3–5 d post partum*
B   Neurotic depression   E   Puerperal psychosis
C   Postnatal depression   *w/in 2 wks*
         2wks – 2mo post partum   *postpartum*

10 A 5-year-old boy has been reported to squirm all the time, unable to sit still in school or home, suffer 'mini accidents' and needs to be spoken to several times or shouted at to catch his attention.

What is the SINGLE most likely diagnosis in this case?

A   ADHD   D   Deafness
B   Autism   E   Learning difficulties
C   Conduct disorder

hyperactivity
inattention
impulsivity

11 A 45-year-old man known to suffer from bipolar affective disorder but who is stable on lithium has recently developed ischaemic heart disease.

Which medications could lead to possible adverse interactions in this condition?

A   ACE inhibitors
B   All of these medications
C   Furosemide
D   NSAIDs and aspirin
E   Thiazide diuretics

12 A 37-year-old woman has been suffering from depression. She has not responded to a trial of paroxetine and then venlafaxine in optimum doses for 6 weeks.

What is the SINGLE best pharmacological option to try at this stage?

A   Add diazepam
B   Add haloperidol
C   Add lithium
D   Try CBT
E   Try ECT

13 A 35-year-old woman admitted to hospital suffering from depression has not responded to a trial of fluoxetine and then amitriptyline at optimum doses.

Which SINGLE combination of investigations might you consider at this stage?

A   Dexamethasone suppression test (DST), urinary drug screen, blood cortisol level
B   DST, urinary drug screen, psychological assessment
C   Thyroid function tests (TFT), DST, blood cortisol level
D   TFT, DST, urinary drug screen
E   TFT, urinary drug screen, psychological assessment

14

Which single drug is UNLIKELY to cause depression as a side-effect?

A   Amoxicillin
B   Digoxin
C   Haloperidol
D   Indometacin
E   Prednisolone

15

Which single antidepressant is NOT commonly associated with 'discontinuation syndrome'?

A   Amitriptyline TCA
B   Fluoxetine
C   Paroxetine

D   Tranylcypromine MAOI
E   Venlafaxine

16 A 25-year-old man with a known history of multiple substance misuse has presented with depression.

Which single antidepressant from the list below would you NOT prescribe in this case?

A   Mirtazapine α₂ blocker
B   Paroxetine
C   Tranylcypromine

D   Trazodone
E   Venlafaxine

17 The parents of a 6-year-old boy with multiple tics are seeking pharmacological help after behavioural management has been of limited assistance.

Which is the SINGLE most appropriate first-line medication in the management of this case?

A   Fluoxetine
B   Haloperidol
C   Lithium

D   Methylphenidate
E   Procyclidine

18 A 76-year-old woman on paroxetine has become increasingly weak and confused.

What is the SINGLE most likely reason for her confusion?

A   Hypercalcaemia
B   Hypernatraemia
C   Hypocalcaemia

D   Hypoglycaemia
E   Hyponatraemia

19

Which of the following conditions have been proved to show benefit from cognitive behavioural therapy?

A   All of these options
B   Chronic fatigue syndrome (CFS)
C   Fibromyalgia
D   Irritable bowel syndrome (IBS)
E   None of these options

20 A 26-year-old man has presented to A&E feeling paranoid, 'hearing' voices and 'seeing' insects. He mentions he has taken 'some drugs'.

Which single substance is he UNLIKELY to have taken? read !

A   Amphetamine
B   Cannabis
C   Cocaine
D   Heroin
E   LSD

21 A 24-year-old mother has brought her 2-year-old son to the hospital with diarrhoea. The staff recognise her from her numerous past visits, which have led to several admissions of the boy and, earlier, his older sister. Both are known to have recovered promptly on admission. She is known to have trained as a nurse.

Which SINGLE option is the most likely?

A   Child abuse
B   Failure to thrive
C   Munchausen syndrome by proxy
D   Non-accidental injury
E   Physical abuse

22 A 76-year-old man is having problems remembering recent events. He is also having difficulty naming objects.

What is the SINGLE most likely diagnosis of the latter phenomenon?

A   Broca's aphasia
B   Communicative aphasia
C   Global aphasia
D   Nominal aphasia
E   Wernicke's aphasia

23 A 37-year-old man is complaining of his inability for the last 3 months to leave his house and travel on his own to work. He also complains of feeling anxious and panic-stricken.

Which is the SINGLE most likely diagnosis?

A   Agoraphobia
B   Anxiety disorder
C   Generalised anxiety disorder
D   Panic attack
E   Social phobia

24 A 43-year-old woman is complaining of several aches, pains and discomfort in her tummy, head and genital region. She has been seen by her GP, and referred to orthopaedics, neurology, gynaecology and gastroenterology units. All investigations were within normal limits and examination revealed no positive findings. However, she continues to suffer and is disabled by the condition.

What is the SINGLE most likely diagnosis?

A   Chronic fatigue syndrome
B   Hypochondriasis
C   Hysteria
D   Neurasthenia
E   Somatoform disorder

25 A 31-year-old single professional man is assessed as he recovers from a serious overdose of 100 paracetamol tablets. He is known to suffer from bipolar affective disorder and is found to be depressed. He has recently discontinued taking lithium. He had jumped off a bridge 3 years ago during a relapse. He manages well on recovery.

What would be the SINGLE best management option at this stage?

A   Detain him under the Mental Health Act
B   Inform the occupational health unit
C   Offer admission
D   Restart his lithium
E   Start him on an antidepressant

Psychiatry SBAs – Answers

1 B: He can resume driving if there is no other complication
A person with uncomplicated depression or anxiety who is stable
on management can return to driving, providing there is no
complication from the medication prescribed, eg medications
with a sedative side-effect. However, fluoxetine is not a sedative
antidepressant. In severe depression or severe anxiety the DVLA
should be informed and driving ceased, pending medical
recommendation (a period of stability is required before driving
can be resumed). In mild dementia the recommendations are
similar but subject to annual review. In cases of acute psychosis or
alcohol or opioid dependency a person's licence is revoked for 12
months and he/she can only resume driving after a drug-free
period of 12 months. Regulations for driving a heavy or public
vehicle are more stringent, and the counterpart of 12 months in
this category is usually 3 years. (Please refer to *www.dvla.gov.uk*
for more detailed information.)

2 D: Have high sensitivity
If there is effective treatment available, highly sensitive tests are
preferred for screening rather than highly specific ones. On the
other hand, for diseases where the treatment is expensive and
painful and has limited efficacy, then more specific tests are
preferred to avoid unnecessary exposure. Exhaustive tests are
never ideal for screening. Internal validity refers to a test
measuring what it set out to measure: it is a generic requirement
of tests and is not specific to screening tools. A reliable test is one
that produces the same result when repeated, and reliability is,
once again, a generic requirement for investigative tests.

3 E: Retrograde amnesia
Following a head injury, the Glasgow Coma Scale score,
post-traumatic amnesia and duration of loss of consciousness are
the most sensitive markers of severity. The duration of
anterograde amnesia is often similar to that of post-traumatic
amnesia. Retrograde amnesia has been shown to be a poor marker
for the severity of closed head injuries.

4   B: **She can be treated with her best interests in mind ('common law')**

The Mental Health Act cannot be used to treat physical illness. To treat this patient under common law, her capacity to consent has to be assessed, which would include her ability to understand and retain information on the options available, and their consequences, and come to a decision and communicate it. Often, simple measures such as calm environment and giving reassurance are helpful in dealing with such situations. Advice from Trust solicitors or defence unions is helpful and can be obtained at the earliest possible opportunity, but it might not be appropriate or available in dealing in with a crisis such as this.

5   A: **He does not know the extent of his belongings**

Other conditions that impede a person's capacity to make a will include not understanding the implications of making a will, not knowing who the possible claimants are, or having a mental condition specifically affecting such judgement.

6   C: **Night terrors**

Somnambulism is sleep-walking and the main concern in its management is safety. Both somnambulism and night terrors are more common in children, occur in non-REM sleep and are known to have a strong familial component. Dreams in the non-REM phase are ill-formed and often not recollected. On the other hand, nightmares occur during REM sleep.

7   C: **Lesch–Nyhan syndrome**

Self-mutilating behaviour is classic in this condition. This syndrome, an X-linked recessive disorder, is caused by an error in purine metabolism, with increased uric acid and xanthine. Tay–Sachs disease is an autosomal recessive gangliosidosis with developmental delay and cherry-red spots on the macula on ophthalmoscopy. Hurler's syndrome is a mucopolysaccharidosis associated with learning disabilities (remember Reilly inclusion bodies in lymphocytes and histiocytes). Prader–Willi syndrome is a chromosome 15-related, paternal-origin deletion presenting as learning disability, hypogonadism and hyperphagia. Maternal origin of same defect produces the Angelman syndrome.

8   B: Down's syndrome

Down's syndrome is more often associated with sociable features rather than autistic ones. Learning disability or autistic features are unlikely in someone with Turner's syndrome but they can be present. Fragile X and tuberous sclerosis carry a high incidence of autism. Asperger's syndrome is similar to autism, although affected individuals have better developed language functions. These conditions are often considered together with autism and Rett's syndrome as 'autistic spectrum disorders' or 'pervasive developmental disorders'.

9   D: Puerperal blues

Mere tearfulness does not warrant a diagnosis of depression and neurotic depression is not a diagnostic category in present usage. Puerperal blues is an extremely common (ie around 50% of postpartum women) condition, occurring within 3–5 days following delivery. Management is primarily reassurance. Between 10% and 15% of postpartum women suffer from postnatal depression (PND), evidenced within 2 weeks to 2 months following delivery. Puerperal psychosis is rare (0.2%), often affective in nature, and seen within 2 weeks of a birth.

10   A: ADHD

ADHD, attention-deficit hyperactivity disorder, is also known as hyperkinetic disorder. The classic triad of symptoms is hyperactivity, inattention and impulsivity. It can be managed with behavioural techniques and medication such as methylphenidate. Autism presents with the triad of social communication difficulties, language problems and deficits in symbolic thinking. All the options are possible and are not mutually exclusive, ie there are high rates of co-morbidity within the conditions, but the most likely diagnosis here is ADHD.

11   B: All of these medications

All of these medications are likely to be prescribed to patients with cardiac conditions, especially hypertension, and all interfere with the renal clearance of lithium and cause its retention, with an increased risk of toxicity. (Refer to the *BNF*.)

12   C: Add lithium

Lithium augmentation is a known and accepted mode of

treatment for resistant depression, ie the scenario described. Electroconvulsive therapy (ECT) or cognitive behavioural therapy (CBT) are effective alternatives but they are not pharmacological options. Benzodiazepines have little role to play in the treatment of resistant depression.

13   E: TFT, urinary drug screen, psychological assessment
Blood cortisol level and DST have little value in current clinical practice for the management of depression.

14   A: Amoxicillin
Digoxin, indometacin, prednisolone and haloperidol can all cause depression.

15   B: Fluoxetine
This is primarily because of its longer half-life. Presentations of the discontinuation syndrome include: flu-like symptoms, shock-like symptoms, dizziness, irritability and increased vivid dreams. Remember the argument for antidepressants not being addictive even though it presents with discontinuation as there is no tolerance.

16   C: Tranylcypromine
Tranylcypromine is partly metabolised to amphetamine and therefore has the potential for abuse.

17   B: Haloperidol
Haloperidol is the only drug licensed in the UK for the treatment of tics (see the *BNF*). Fluoxetine can be used as a second-line agent. Methylphenidate is known to exacerbate tics, while procyclidine and lithium have no effect.

18   E: Hyponatraemia

Risk factors for antidepressant-induced hyponatraemia include old age, female sex, low body weight, co-morbidity and polypharmacy. Dizziness, nausea, cramps, confusion, lethargy and, in severe cases, seizures may result from hyponatraemia.

19   A: All of these options
CFS, IBS and fibromyalgia all are similar disorders, in the sense that their aetiology is not clearly known. The conditions have been shown to respond to psychological interventions such as

CBT. However, it is believed there is a physiological as well as a psychological contribution to these conditions.

20 D: Heroin

Apart from heroin, any of these substances may result in psychotic experiences such as hallucinations and delusions.

21 C: Munchausen syndrome by proxy

While it is true that this can be classified as non-accidental injury and physical/child abuse, a presentation such as the one described is unique (and rare) and known as 'Munchausen syndrome by proxy'. This syndrome manifests as repeated presentations by a parent complaining that their child is ill. At times, the illness is induced or fabricated. An adult similarly presenting her/himself has 'Munchausen syndrome', which is considered a factitious illness, with no obvious gain (cf malingering). This is a serious and rare matter, and should be dealt with sensitively with child protection in mind.

22 D: Nominal aphasia

Broca's aphasia is motor aphasia with paucity of speech, eg telegraphic speech. It is associated with a frontal motor lesion. Wernicke's aphasia is a sensory aphasia, whereby the affected person speaks fluently without making sense – 'jargon aphasia' (associated with a parietal lobe lesion). Communicative aphasia presents with an inability to repeat words and is associated with a lesion in the arcuate fasciculus. Global aphasia is relatively common and is associated with a gross lesion in the brain. Nominal aphasia is seen in early dementia, particularly of the Alzheimer's type, which might in later stages progress to global aphasia.

23 A: Agoraphobia

The main complaints of people with agoraphobia are of experiencing panic while on their own, travelling alone or being away from home. It is often associated with panic attacks. If the attacks are not limited to a fear/situation, then a diagnosis of panic attack should be considered. Social phobia sufferers may also present with an inability to leave their home, but their fear is of facing people and being criticised or embarrassed. All the options can be considered under the rubric of 'anxiety disorder', which is not a diagnostic category in its own right in current classification systems.

24 E: Somatoform disorder

In the case of hypochondriasis the patient is extremely worried about a particular diagnosis, and is not reassured. Neurasthenia is a controversial diagnosis similar to chronic fatigue syndrome: CFS is retained in ICD-10. CFS is a more specific diagnosis, presenting with recent-onset fatigue, lymph node swelling, joint pain, etc and is being researched by both physicians and psychiatrists. Historically, hysteria was thought to be associated with somatoform disorders, but this is not a view generally accepted today. It is no longer a diagnosis retained in recent classifications, and is instead considered under dissociative or conversion disorders.

25 C: Offer admission

While all the options are possibilities, his immediate management should involve admission, followed by reinstating his medication. Occupational health (OH) can be contacted, with his consent, at a later date: it is useful to involve OH when planning his return to work. If he refuses admission then Mental Health Act assessment might be considered, but it is always preferable to work with the patient and there is no indication in this scenario that he is refusing to accept help.

Part 2

Practice Paper

Practice Paper Questions

Theme: **Cirrhosis of the liver**

Options

A   α₁-Antitrypsin deficiency
B   Cryptogenic cirrhosis
C   Haemochromatosis   A ᴅ
D   Hepatocellular carcinoma
E   Indian childhood cirrhosis

F   Infectious mononucleosis
G   Lupoid hepatitis
H   Primary biliary cirrhosis
I   Sarcoidosis of the liver
J   Wilson's disease   A ᴿ

Instructions

For each of the patients described below choose the SINGLE most appropriate diagnosis from the list of options above. Each option may be used once, more than once or not at all.

1 A 52-year-old man complained of increasing breathlessness, fatigue and pain in the knees. He also complained of recent-onset impotence. Liver function tests were abnormal. ☐

2 A 38-year-old man with a 20-pack-year history of smoking presented with increasing breathlessness. He was found to have an obstructive pattern on spirometry. He was admitted to hospital when he presented with melaena. *bleeding d/t liver dse* ☐

3 A 40-year-old man with jaundice and ankle swelling developed tremor and poor co-ordination. He was also noted to have speech problems. ☐

4 A 24-year-old lady presented generally unwell and jaundiced. She had amenorrhoea. She then developed epistaxis and bleeding gums and began to bruise easily. ☐

5 A 45-year-old lady comes to you complaining of generalised pruritus for the last 6 months. On examination, you find excoriation marks over the extensor aspects of her hands, legs and body. ☐

6 A 26-year-old primigravida developed HELLP syndrome at 32 weeks of pregnancy. Which is the SINGLE most characteristic abnormal report among the following blood tests that is consistent with this diagnosis?

A   Alkaline phosphatase 120 U/l
B   Aspartate transaminase (AST) 32 U/l
C   Haemoglobin 8.5 g/dl
D   Platelet count 60 × 10⁹/l
E   Serum bilirubin 7 µmol/l

7 A 62-year-old man has an oesophegectomy for cancer and then develops an anastomotic leak, sepsis, and respiratory failure for which he needs long-term ventilation. It is decided that he needs total parenteral nutrition (TPN). Which ONE of the following statements about TPN is true?

A   Catheter-induced sepsis is mainly caused by Gram-negative cocci
B   Electrolytes should be checked weekly *daily*
C   Heparin is added to the solution
D   Hypoglycaemia is a recognised complication
E   Nitrogen balance should be checked daily *weekly*

Theme: **Multiple trauma diagnosis**

Options

A   Aortic rupture
B   Cardiac tamponade
C   Flail chest
D   Intracranial bleeding
E   Ruptured bronchus
F   Ruptured chordae tendinae of the mitral valve
G   Ruptured oesophagus
H   Tension pneumothorax

Instructions

For each of the patients described below choose the SINGLE most appropriate diagnosis from the list of options above. Each option may be used once, more than once or not at all.

8 A 50-year-old taxi driver was brought to A&E after a head-on collision with another car at 50 km/hour (80 mph). Initially thought to be stable, it was noticed shortly afterwards that he had started to deteriorate. Chest X-rays reveal a widened mediastinum. □

9 A 61-year-old man fell from a 3.6-m- (12-ft-) high ladder and landed on the back of his head. He has been brought unconscious into A&E and is found to have a dilated right pupil. □

10 A man with multiple injuries was taken to theatre for reduction of an open tibial fracture. During the operation the anaesthetist notices that his oxygen saturation has dropped, with tachycardia and hypotension, associated with a rise in ventilation pressure. □

11 A 24-year-old man who was driving a car without a seatbelt was involved in an RTA. His chest hit the steering wheel. In A&E he was found to have a right-sided pneumothorax, a collapsed lung and pneumomediastinum on chest X-ray. A chest drain was inserted but his condition has not improved. □

12 A 20-year-old man was involved in an RTA and brought to A&E. He has difficulty breathing and his chest is bruised due to a steering-wheel injury. A segment of the right side of the chest seems to be moving with respiration. □

---

13 A 36-year-old woman regularly consumes around 40 units of alcohol per week. Which ONE of the following statements is true?

A 20% of people who regularly drink alcohol develop liver cirrhosis
B Alcohol dehydrogenase is most prevalent in the small intestine
C 'Hangover' after drinking is a neurotoxic effect of alcohol
D Occasional binges are more harmful than regular heavy drinking
E Pregnant women should abstain only in the first trimester □

---

14 Which ONE of the following conditions has an X-linked dominant pattern of inheritance?

A Achondroplasia *AD*   D Phenylketonuria *AR*
B Colour blindness *XR*   E Vitamin D-resistant rickets
C Haemophilia *X R* □

Theme: **Skin disorders**

Options

A	Bullous pemphigoid	F	Pemphigus vulgaris
B	Dermatitis herpetiformis	G	Pompholyx
C	Guttate psoriasis	H	Porphyria cutanea tarda
D	Lichen planus	I	Seborrhoeic dermatitis
E	Micropapular sarcoid	J	Stevens–Johnson syndrome

Instructions

For each of the patients described below choose the SINGLE most appropriate diagnosis from the list of options above. Each option may be used once, more than once or not at all.

15 A 10-year-old boy developed very small scaly patches of skin over the trunk and limbs. The rash followed a throat infection. ☐

16 A 38-year-old man was prescribed ferrous sulphate tablets by his GP. He developed small fluid-filled blisters on the back of his hands and face. The skin became easily bruised. Scarring and small white skin cysts developed. The lesions were only in the sun-exposed parts of the body. ☐

17 A 35-year-old lady with a low BMI and regular bouts of diarrhoea developed itchy, red, raised patches and small blisters affecting the knees and elbows. ☐

18 A 46-year-old man who was put on chloroquine tablets for malaria prophylaxis developed purple-coloured areas of fissured skin on the flexor surfaces of the forearms and the back of his neck. ☐

19 A 28-year-old man comes to his GP with painful swelling in the axillas. On examination, you notice discharging pustules, papules and generalised scaly erythematous lesions over the axillas and the trunk. ☐

20 A 71-year-old man with extensive bladder tumour (and involvment as far as the muscle layer) is admitted with recurrent haematuria. Previously, he has received both radiotherapy and chemotherapy. What is the SINGLE best treatment?

A   Ileal conduit   D   Radical cystectomy
B   Intravesical chemotherapy   E   Salvage cystectomy
C   Palliative treatment

---

21 A 42-year-old lady is diagnosed with ulcerative colitis. Which ONE
of the following statements about the medical management of
ulcerative colitis is true?

A   In severe ulcerative colitis, patients who do not respond to high-dose
intravenous steroids may respond to azathioprine
B   Moderate attacks may conveniently be treated with local rectal
steroids in the form of an enema
C   Patients in a clinical remission, with no relapses, can usually stop
sulfasalazine after 1 symptom-free year
D   Patients with a severe attack are best treated with sulfasalazine
E   Severe attacks of ulcerative colitis usually carry a mortality rate of
< 1% when treated in a hospital

Theme: **Infectious disease in pregnancy**

Options

A   Congenital cytomegalovirus   G   Hepatitis C
B   Congenital rubella   H   Herpes hominis   HSV 2
C   Congenital syphilis   I   HIV
D   Congenital toxoplasmosis   J   Listeriosis   + ampicillin + genta
E   Fetal varicella syndrome   K   Parvovirus infection
F   Hepatitis B

+f. Spiramycin

Instructions

*For each of the clinical signs described below choose the SINGLE most
appropriate causative factor from the list of options given above. Each
option may be used once, more than once or not at all.*

22 While doing a home visit you notice vesicular pustular lesions on
the scalp of a 16-day-old neonate. The infant also has red, swollen,
watery eyes and yellow skin. On examination, you notice mild
hepatomegaly.

23 While performing a 20-weeks anomaly scan on a high-risk pregnant woman you notice hydrocephalus with cerebral calcification. ☐

24 A 26-year-old 34-weeks pregnant woman presents to the labour ward with flu-like symptoms and diarrhoea. She also complains of not having felt the baby move since yesterday. A scan confirms intrauterine death. She is induced and delivers a macerated fetus. The placenta shows multiple abscesses. ☐

25 A mother brings her 18-month-old child to the paediatric unit. He has diarrhoea and vomiting. On examination, you notice the child to be grossly emaciated with generalised lymphadenopathy. You also notice that he has hepatosplenomegaly and parotitis. While taking a history, you gather that the family has recently emigrated from West Africa. ☐

26 A 2-year-old boy is referred by the GP to the paediatric unit with a high temperature and signs suggestive of meningitis. On general physical examination, you notice 'snuffles' and Hutchinson's teeth. ☐

---

27 A 56-year-old man was brought into A&E after suddenly collapsing. Which ONE of the following statements is correct?

A   A history of nausea, vomiting and diarrhoea, associated with hypertension, hypoglycaemia and hypokalaemia are consistent with an addisonian crisis   ↑Na ↓K

B   Pallor and unresponsiveness during the collapse, followed by facial flushing and rapid recovery suggest transient bradyarrhythmia as a cause

C   Palpitations, profuse sweating, hypertension and syncope are characteristic features of severe thyrotoxicosis

D   Sharp pleuritic chest pain and severe breathlessness suggest pulmonary embolism, and a high D-dimer level would establish the diagnosis

E   Twitching limb movements lasting around 30 seconds strongly suggest epilepsy ☐

28 A 32-year-old bus driver, who has recovered from a manic episode while taking sodium valproate, continues to drive against medical advice. As the psychiatrist responsible for his care what is your SINGLE best option?

A   Can use your discretion to inform the DVLA
B   Cannot inform the DVLA due to confidentiality
C   Discuss with his wife
D   Inform the DVLA
E   Should inform the police

Theme: **AIDS-related ocular problems**

Options

A   Acute retinal necrosis syndrome
B   CMV retinitis
C   Kaposi's sarcoma of the conjunctiva
D   Orbital lymphoma
E   *Pneumocystis carinii* choroiditis
F   Progressive outer retinal necrosis syndrome
G   Syphilitic anterior and posterior uveitis
H   *Toxoplasma gondii* chorioretinitis
I   Tuberculous choroiditis

Instructions

For each of the patients described below choose the SINGLE most appropriate diagnosis from the list of options above. Each option may be used once, more than once or not at all.

29 A 26-year-old man developed headache and personality changes, and then grand mal seizures. This was followed by retinal scarring and blindness.

30 A patient with AIDS and a CD4 count of 75 developed a polyradiculopathy known as the 'cauda equina syndrome'. Ocular examination showed features of retinitis. The early lesion appeared as small yellow-white patches with a grainy appearance, often with accompanying bleeding.

pizza eye appearance - CMV

31 A 75-year-old man with known HIV of 3 years' duration developed chronic haemorrhagic thickening of the conjunctiva. Although surgically unresectable, the conjunctival lesion responded satisfactorily to radiotherapy. ☐

32 A 56-year-old HIV-positive man developed mediastinal lymphadenopathy followed by proptosis. ☐

33 A 45-year-old HIV-positive man with generalised wasting and jaundice comes to you complaining of misting of vision, with red and painful eyes. ☐

---

34 A 7-year-old child is diagnosed with a Colles' fracture. You plan to reduce it with the help of a Bier's block. Which one of the following anaesthetic agents is the SINGLE most suitable medication in this case?

A   Benzocaine
B   Bupivacaine – cardiotoxic
C   Lidocaine with adrenaline (epinephrine)
D   Mercaine
E   Prilocaine ☐

35 A 28-year-old man presented to A&E with palpitations and chest pain. His ECG showed an SVT. The rate was controlled and subsequent examination revealed a double apical impulse, and an audible fourth heart sound and an ejection systolic murmur which was increased by the Valsalva manoeuvre. The ECG showed left ventricular hypertrophy with right bundle branch block, widespread ST-segment and T-wave changes. Which pulse character should be sought in this condition?

A   Anacrotic pulse AS   D   Pulsus bisferiens
B   Pulsus alternans   E   Pulsus paradoxus
C   Pulsus bigeminus ☐

pathognomonic of
HOCM

Theme: **Febrile children with rashes**

Options

A	Chickenpox	F	Measles 3 Cs
B	Erythema infectiosum	G	Meningococcal meningitis
C	Glandular fever	H	Mumps
D	Hand, foot and mouth disease	I	Rubella
E	Kawasaki disease	J	Scarlet fever

Instructions

For each of the patients described below choose the SINGLE most appropriate diagnosis from the list of options above. Each option may be used once, more than once or not at all.

36 A 4-year-old child with a history of fever, headache and myalgia has developed a characteristic rash on both cheeks. □

37 A 3-year-old girl presents with a history of a high temperature for 5 days, conjunctivitis, swollen neck glands and cracked lips. □

38 A 4-year-old child with mild fever and arthralgia presents with a maculopapular rash that started on her face and has spread centrifugally. On examination, she has swollen postauricular and suboccipital glands. □

39 A 5-year-old child with a fever and headache develops a vesicular rash all over his body and inside his mouth. □

40 A 7-month-old baby is brought in with a high temperature, poor feeding, irritability and a rapidly spreading rash. □

41 A 46-year-old lady on long-term treatment for psychiatric problems developed polyuria and polydipsia. Osmolality results revealed nephrogenic diabetes insipidus. There was also chronic renal impairment, a raised TSH level and a leucocytosis. Which ONE of the following is the most likely agent which might be responsible?

A	Clonidine	D	Risperidone
B	Clozapine	E	Trazodone
C	Lithium		

□

42 A 24-year-old man known to suffer from epilepsy has recently been expressing low mood with hopelessness. His GP is concerned about the risk of inducing seizures by prescribing an antidepressant. Which of the following medications is the SINGLE best option in this case?

A   Amitriptyline
B   Bupropion
C   Fluoxetine

D   Moclobemide   MAOI
E   Venlafaxine

☐

Theme: **Pleural effusion**

Options

A   Hypothyroidism
B   Lymphoma
C   Meigs' syndrome
D   Mesothelioma
E   Pulmonary infarction

F   Rheumatoid arthritis
G   Sarcoidosis
H   SLE
I   Tuberculosis

Instructions

For each of the patients described below choose the SINGLE most appropriate diagnosis from the list of options above. Each option may be used once, more than once or not at all.

43 A 64-year-old man with known metastatic prostatic carcinoma presented with sudden-onset shortness of breath and small amounts of streaky haemoptysis.   ☐

44 A 72-year-old smoker presented with gradually increasing shortness of breath and dull, aching chest pain. A CT scan of his chest showed pleural thickening and a pleural effusion.   ☐

45 A 36-year-old woman with small-joint polyarthralgia and proteinuria was found to have a pleuropericardial effusion.   ☐

46 A 38-year-old lady with generalised tiredness and lethargy, menorrhagia, and a coarse, dry skin was found to have a pleural effusion on her chest X-ray.   ☐

47 A 34-year-old man from Eastern Europe comes to his GP with chronic cough and occasional dyspnoea. The chest X-ray shows nodular shadows in the upper zone.   ☐

48 You are counselling a 35-year-old pregnant woman. Which ONE of the following represents the risk of her having a baby with Down's syndrome?

A   1 in 40   D   1 in 380
B   1 in 100   E   1 in 900
C   1 in 249

---

49 A 40-year-old man with a family history of mucosal neuroma presented with a firm thyroid mass, cough and diarrhoea. Clinical examination revealed enlarged cervical lymph nodes. A thyroid scan showed a cold nodule. The calcitonin level was found to be substantially higher than normal. What is the SINGLE most likely diagnosis?

A   Anaplastic carcinoma of the thyroid
B   Follicular carcinoma of the thyroid
C   Medullary carcinoma of the thyroid
D   Papillary carcinoma of the thyroid
E   Riedel's thyroiditis

Theme: **Hip fractures**

Options

A   Austin Moore hemiarthroplasty   F   Skeletal traction
B   Cannulated screws   G   Skin traction
C   Distal condylar screws   H   Spiral blade
D   Dynamic hip screw   I   Thomas splint
E   Intramedullary nail

Instructions

For each of the patients described below choose the SINGLE most appropriate management from the list of options above. Each option may be used once, more than once or not at all.

50 A 91-year-old woman presents to A&E with an intracapsular fracture of the neck of the femur.

51 A 75-year-old man presents with an intertrochanteric fracture of the neck of the femur. ☐

52 A 55-year-old woman presents to A&E after a fall at home when she landed awkwardly on her left hip. She has rheumatoid arthritis. ☐

53 A 34-year-old man was brought to A&E after a car crash. His ABC was normal. However, his left leg is found to be shortened and externally rotated. *displaced femoral neck fx* ☐

54 A 56-year-old man has sustained an infratrochanteric fracture of the femur in an RTA. ☐

---

55 A 62-year-old man was referred to the neurology department with suspected dementia. He has suffered increasing memory problems over the past 9 months, and more recently has been noted to suffer episodes of ataxia and incontinence. A lumbar puncture showed opening pressures in the high-normal range, and CSF microscopy was normal. The patient was noted to have improved gait and cognition after the lumbar puncture. What is the most likely diagnosis?

A   Depression
B   Huntington's disease
C   Normal-pressure hydrocephalus
D   Parkinson's disease
E   Thiamine deficiency ☐

---

56 A 30-year-old lady comes to the gynaecological clinic, referred by the GP in view of her family history of ovarian and breast cancer. Both her mother and her sister had developed breast cancer by the age of 40. Which is the SINGLE most important gene that will explain this hereditary link?

A   *ABL-1*
B   *BCL-2*
C   *BRCA1*
D   *RCA3*
E   *MYC* ☐

Theme: **Spastic paraparesis**

Options

A   Anterior spinal artery thrombosis
B   Familial spastic paraparesis
C   Friedreich's ataxia
D   Motor neurone disease
E   Multiple sclerosis

F   Subacute combined
    degeneration of the cord
G   Syringomyelia
H   Tabes dorsalis
I   Tropical spastic paraplegia
J   von Recklinghausen's disease

Instructions

For each of the patients described below choose the SINGLE most appropriate diagnosis from the list of options above. Each option may be used once, more than once or not at all.

57 A 26-year-old man presented to his GP complaining of pain in the upper limbs that was exacerbated by coughing and exertion. Examination revealed loss of pain and temperature sensation but not of light touch. There was loss of reflexes in the upper limbs. ☐

58 A 36-year-old man developed bacterial endocarditis secondary to his rheumatic valvular heart disease. This was being treated in hospital when he suddenly developed acute-onset paraplegia. ☐

59 A 62-year-old man developed difficulty in swallowing, followed by frequent aspiration of food. Examination revealed weakness and wasting of the small muscles of the hand. ☐

60 A 56-year-old man with a known malabsorption syndrome presented with tingling and numbness in the feet. There was weakness and wasting in the legs and he had an unsteady gait. ☐

61 A 42-year-old man comes to his GP complaining of severe headache and visual disturbances for the last few weeks. He has also recently noticed weakness in his right leg. You notice him to have several small macules on his face. His blood pressure is 180/120 mmHg in the clinic. ☐

62 A 55-year-old man who is on warfarin presents with a massive haematemesis. What is the SINGLE best product to use in cases of warfarin over-anticoagulation in the emergency situation?

A   Fresh frozen plasma   D   Platelets
B   Factor VIII extract   E   Whole blood
C   Factor X extract

---

63 A 48-year-old woman was referred for investigation of jaundice, and a number of biochemical tests were requested. Which ONE of the following statements is true?

A   A low albumin concentration can indicate cirrhosis or cancer
B   Cholestasis is typically associated with a greater rise in alanine aminotransferase (ALT) than alkaline phosphatase (ALP)
C   Cholestatic jaundice is a recognised complication of ingesting Jamaican bush tea
D   Failure of prothrombin time to correct after intravenous vitamin K usually indicates biliary obstruction
E   High ALP concentrations characteristically indicate hepatocellular injury

---

Theme: **Appropriate psychotherapy**

Options

A   Analytical psychotherapy   F   Dialectic behaviour therapy
B   Behaviour therapy   G   Family therapy
C   Cognitive behaviour therapy   H   Interpersonal therapy
D   Cognitive therapy   I   Psychodynamic psychotherapy
E   Counselling   J   Reality-orientation therapy

Instructions

For each of the patients described below choose the SINGLE most appropriate psychotherapy from the list of options above. Each option may be used once, more than once or not at all.

64 An 11-year-old boy who was referred from school for being disruptive and difficult in class has been assessed, and it is felt

unlikely to be ADHD. However, his parents are undergoing an
acrimonious divorce. ☐

65 A 19-year-old girl has been diagnosed to be suffering from mild to
moderate anorexia nervosa. She moved to London from her home
in Leeds last year and is sharing a flat with her friend. ☐

66 A 40-year-old banker is having recurrent and distressing thoughts
of harming children. He is both scared and ashamed of himself.
He has never acted on these thoughts and, after suffering for
6 months, is now seeking help. ☐

67 An 83-year-old World War II veteran is living alone after his wife
died. He has been diagnosed with mild dementia and is on
cholinesterase inhibitors. He has day-care and meals-on-wheels
support. ☐

68 A 15-year-old boy with a moderate learning disability who is
attending a 'special school' presents with challenging behaviour. ☐

---

69 A 2-year-old boy has been brought to A&E following a fall and his
knees are severely bruised. His parents say that they have noticed
that he has always bruised severely, and has continued to bleed for
longer than usual following a minor injury. The history of the
accident is consistent with examination of the child and there are
no concerns regarding non-accidental injury. Which SINGLE
statement below pertains to this child's condition?

A   Desmopressin is the treatment of choice for people undergoing
surgery or in cases of major life-threatening bleeding
B   It commonly presents with bleeding into muscles and joints
C   It has an X-linked dominant pattern of inheritance
D   It is characterised by reduced or absent factor XI activity
E   The prothrombin time is elevated, while the APTT (activated partial
thromboplastin time) is normal ☐

Ⓝ PT   ↑ aPTT

70 A 62-year-old man presented to A&E with confusion and altered conscious level. He was found to have a serum sodium concentration of 127 mmol/l (normal range 137–144 mmol/l). Which ONE of the following statements is true about hyponatraemia?

A   Adrenal insufficiency is associated with reduced ADH secretion
B   Hyponatraemia in the setting of heart failure is due to increased circulating volume and decreased ADH levels
C   In psychogenic polydipsia there is an element of renal impairment which leads to hyponatraemia
D   Mannitol is a recognised cause of SIADH
E   SIADH usually occurs due to non-physiological release of ADH from the posterior pituitary or an ectopic source ☐

---

71 A 26-year-old man who has just come back from the tropics complains of bloody diarrhoea with mucus, and pain in the right hypochondrium. Which is the SINGLE most likely diagnosis?

A   Amoebic colitis
B   Bacterial colitis
C   Diverticular disease
D   Ischaemic colitis
E   Typhoid fever ☐

Theme: **Ptosis**

Options

A   Dystrophia myotonica
B   Horner's syndrome
C   Mitochondrial myopathy
D   Myasthenia gravis
E   Orbital tumour
F   Pancoast's tumour
G   Syringomyelia
H   Tabes dorsalis
I   Third nerve palsy

Instructions

For each of the patients described below choose the SINGLE most appropriate diagnosis from the list of options above. Each option may be used once, more than once or not at all.

72 A 48-year-old man, known to be HIV-positive, developed weakness, diminished reflexes, unsteady gait and bilateral ptosis.

There was progressive degeneration of the joints and loss of co-ordination. He also developed personality changes, dementia and deafness. ☐

73 A 19-year-old man was found to have progressive muscle weakness and exercise intolerance. He experienced seizures and transient ischaemic attacks. He developed droopy eyelids and limited mobility of his eyes, followed by deafness and movement disorders. ☐

74 A 42-year-old woman presented with weakness of proximal muscles and droopiness of the eyelids. Direct questioning revealed fatiguability in speech and mastication. ☐

75 A 40-year-old man had progressive distal muscle weakness, ptosis and thinning of the face. He had diminution of vision due to cataracts. He presented to the hospital with heart failure, which was later found to be due to cardiomyopathy. ☐

76 A 30-year-old-man comes to his GP complaining of sudden onset of ptosis. He recently underwent surgery for removal of a thyroid nodule. ☐

---

77 A 4-year-old girl was brought to the clinic having suffered from recurrent episodes of sore throat, which did not improve with antibiotics. She was tired and lethargic and looked pale. Her parents have noticed that she bruises more easily and has had a temperature on most days over the last few weeks. On examination, she had pallor and hepatosplenomegaly. A full blood count showed a low haemoglobin, high WCC and low platelets, and the peripheral film revealed the presence of blast cells. Which SINGLE statement below best relates to the suspected condition?

A   It has very poor prognosis
B   It is the commonest childhood malignancy
C   It usually presents with a sudden onset of symptoms
D   Median age of occurrence is 9 years
E   Poor prognostic markers are female gender, Caucasian origin, WCC $< 100 \times 10^9/l$ ☐

---

78 A 52-year-old man was diagnosed with obstructive sleep apnoea (OSA) syndrome. Which ONE of the following statements about the management of this condition is true?

A   Acetazolamide is considered to be an effective treatment in mild to moderate OSA

B   Continuous positive airway pressure (CPAP) is useful only in OSA and not in central sleep apnoea

C   In patients with ischaemic heart disease and OSA, nasal CPAP is considered the treatment of choice

D   Intra-oral devices are effective in a minority of patients

E   Uvulopalatopharyngoplasty is effective in more than 90% of patients with OSA ☐

Theme: **Teratogenicity**

Options

A	Alcohol	G	Phenytoin
B	Aminoglycosides	H	Sodium valproate
C	Diethylstilbestrol	I	Tetracycline
D	Glucucorticoids	J	Thalidomide
E	Indometacin	K	Warfarin
F	Norethisterone		

Instructions

For each of the clinical signs described below choose the SINGLE most appropriate causative factor from the list of options given above. Each option may be used once, more than once or not at all.

79 Cleft lip, cardiac anomalies and skeletal defects. ☐

80 Nasal hypoplasia, chondrodysplasia punctata and CNS abnormalities. ☐

81 Microcephaly, facial abnormalities, growth retardation. ☐

82 Premature closure of the ductus arteriosus. ☐

83 Adenocarcinoma of the vagina in the female offspring. ☐

84 A 50-year-old lady was found to have proteinuria on dipstick urinalysis examination. Which ONE of the following statements is true?

A   Most glomerulonephritides (except minimal-change) will predominantly cause selective loss of albumin
B   Normal individuals can excrete up to 150 g of protein per day
C   Plasma-cell dyscrasia may cause a large volume of protein loss which may not be picked up by dipstick urinalysis
D   The degree of oedema does not correlate with the degree of proteinuria
E   Total daily excretion of protein exceeding 3.5 g is always associated with hyperlipidaemia

---

85 A 46-year-old man comes to your clinic complaining of severe pain and difficulty in defecation. On examination, you confirm the diagnosis and put him on the waiting list for surgery. In which ONE of these conditions does Goodsall's rule apply?

A   Anal carcinoma   D   Perianal abscess
B   Fissure-in-ano   E   Rectal carcinoma
C   Fistula-in-ano

Theme: **Congenital heart disease**

Options

A   ASD   F   PDA
B   Coarctation of the aorta   G   Pulmonary stenosis
C   Double aortic arch   H   Transposition of the great arteries
D   Ebstein's anomaly   I   VSD
E   Fallot's tetralogy

Instructions

For each of the patients described below choose the SINGLE most appropriate diagnosis from the list of options above. Each option may be used once, more than once or not at all.

86 A 4-year-old child with Turner's syndrome was found to have weak pulses in the foot.

87 A 27-year-old man presented to the cardiologist with palpitations. Clinical examination revealed additional heart sounds. ECG revealed Wolff–Parkinson–White syndrome. ☐

88 A 12-month-old baby presented with recurrent episodes of deep cyanosis and possible syncope. Physical signs included a sustained parasternal heave and a systolic ejection murmur. ☐

89 A 6-month-old baby presented with stridor and difficulty in swallowing. A barium swallow demonstrated narrowing of the oesophagus. ☐

90 A newborn baby had to be transferred to the SCBU (special care baby unit) within a few hours of his birth, as he became progressively more and more breathless and cyanotic. An arterial blood gas analysis showed the baby to be severely acidotic. ☐

---

91 A 5-year-old boy was brought by his mother to see the GP with mild fever, pain in his joints, which moved from one to another, and malaise over the past few weeks. He had suffered from a sore throat about 3 weeks earlier. Which SINGLE investigation would best confirm the diagnosis?

A	ASO titre	D	Full blood count
B	ECG	E	MSU
C	ESR		

☐

---

92 A 26-year-old man had a splenectomy for traumatic splenic rupture. Which ONE of the following is true of the postsplenectomy period?

A Gram-negative enterococci are the most common organisms causing infection in splenectomised patients

B Pneumococcal vaccine should be administered 2 weeks after elective splenectomy

C Routine chemoprophylaxis with oral penicillin is recommended

D The immediate postsplenectomy period is characterised by thrombocytopenia and leucopenia ✗

E There is no increased incidence of viral infections ☐

Theme: **Postoperative complications**

Options

A	Acute tubular necrosis (ATN)	G	Pelvic abscess
B	Chest infection	H	Pulmonary embolus (PE)
C	Congestive cardiac failure (CCF)	I	Septicaemia
D	Deep vein thrombosis (DVT)	J	Transfusion reaction
E	Impending wound dehiscence	K	Urinary retention
F	Myocardial infarction (MI)	L	Wound infection

Instructions

For each of the patients described below choose the SINGLE most likely complication from the list of options above. Each option may be used once, more than once or not at all.

93 A 49-year-old woman had an anterior resection 1week ago. She now complains of left calf pain and swelling. She has mild pyrexia, with a tender left calf and pitting oedema. ☐

94 A 72-year-old man who has undergone an AAA repair presents with a very low urine output postoperatively. His BP is stable. ☐

95 A 61-year-old woman had a laparotomy for investigation of peritonitis. Postoperatively she has a temperature of 38.4 °C and is hypotensive. ☐

96 A 54-year-old man has just had a hernia operation and is in the recovery room when he is found to be very restless despite an otherwise smooth recovery. There seems to be a swelling in his lower abdomen. ☐

97 A 68-year-old man underwent a total cystectomy. During the first postoperative night he was not producing a satisfactory urine output despite adequate hydration. You involved a senior colleague and, after adequate resuscitation, the patient's urine output slowly picked up. Now, the following day, he is showing evidence of diuresis. ☐

98 A 65-year-old man presented with fever, weight loss and anorexia. Later he was investigated for easy bruising, and was diagnosed with acute myeloid leukaemia (AML). Which ONE of the following statements about AML subtypes is true?

A   Bleeding associated with DIC is common in the M3 subtype
B   Gum infiltration occurs in the M4 and M5 subtypes   *M5*
C * Intracranial haemorrhage is commonest in the M5 subtype
D   Renal tubular dysfunction may be common in the M3 subtype
E   The M4 subtype is associated with a chromosome 15:17 translocation   *M3*   *B*

---

99 A 37-year-old Asian man presents with an ulcer on his shin which has undermined edges. What is the SINGLE most likely diagnosis?

A   Aphthous ulcer   D   Tuberculous ulcer
B   Ischaemic ulcer   E   Venous ulcer
C   Neuropathic ulcer

---

100 A 32-year-old woman went to her GP enquiring about vaccination in relation to pregnancy. Which ONE of the following statements is correct?

A   Inactivated vaccines like HBV and influenza are contraindicated in pregnancy
B   Infants born to mothers vaccinated for rubella in pregnancy have a high risk of congenital rubella syndrome
C   Polio and yellow fever vaccines are the only live virus vaccines which are contraindicated in pregnancy   *MMR*
D   Pregnant women can safely receive tetanus and diphtheria toxoids
E   Women not vaccinated in childhood should be vaccinated with mumps, measles and rubella vaccine

---

Live – MMR polio (sabin), yellow fever

Theme: **Autoantibodies in collagen vascular diseases**

Options

A	ANF	F	Anti-Ro antibody	*Sjögren*
B	Anticardiolipin antibody	G	Anti-Scl-70 antibody	*Scleroder...*
C	Anti-dsDNA	H	LE cells	
D	Antihistone antibody	I	VDRL-positive	
E	Anti-Jo-1 antibody			

drug-induced lupus

Polymyo, dermatomyositis

Instructions

For each of the patients described below choose the SINGLE most appropriate investigation finding from the list of options above. Each option may be used once, more than once or not at all.

101 A 40-year-old lady presented with progressive weakness. Lung function tests showed diaphragmatic weakness. There was also a purple discoloration around the eyes and periorbital oedema. ☐

102 A 36-year-old lady presented with dryness of the mouth and dyspareunia. Chest X-ray showed interstitial shadowing and reduction of lung volume. ☐

103 A 32-year-old lady had recurrent transient ischaemic attacks, followed by right-sided hemiparesis. Blood tests showed thrombocytopenia. She was also found to have livedo reticularis ☐

104 A 17-year-old girl developed a tubercular pleural effusion. She developed a photosensitive rash over her face and vasculitic lesions along the fingertips.   *SLE* ☐

105 A 45-year-old woman went to her GP complaining of difficulty in swallowing for the last 6 months. Recently she has also noticed that she is having difficulty in fully opening her mouth. ☐

106 A 36-year-old woman, who lives with her supportive husband, has become increasing psychotic following the birth of their third child. She is found to be depressed with psychotic symptoms, she is refusing food and medication and believes her baby to be evil. After her admission, what would be the SINGLE most appropriate immediate management option?

A   Consider cognitive behaviour therapy
B   Consider ECT
C   Discharge her into the community and treat with fluoxetine
D   Inform Social Services for protection of the child
E   Transfer to the mother and baby unit

107 A 26-year-old woman developed a high fever and vomiting on the third day of her period. She then developed a macular erythematous rash over her face and trunk, associated with confusion, conjunctival suffusion, peripheral oedema and a strawberry-like appearance of her tongue. What is the most likely diagnosis?

A   Stevens–Johnson syndrome   D   Typhoid fever
B   Toxic epidermal necrolysis   E   Yellow fever
C   Toxic shock syndrome

Theme: **Chromosomal abnormalities**

Options

A   DiGeorge syndrome   F   Noonan's syndrome
B   Down's syndrome   G   Patau's syndrome
C   Edward's syndrome   H   Pierre Robin syndrome
D   Fragile X syndrome   I   Prader–Willi syndrome
E   Klinefelter's syndrome   J   Turner's syndrome
        gynecomastia

Instructions

For each of the patients described below choose the SINGLE most appropriate diagnosis from the list of options above. Each option may be used once, more than once or not at all.

108 A child with a short philtrum, thin upper lip and prominent ears presents with respiratory distress and a heart murmur. Investigations reveal an interrupted aortic arch and a ventricular septal defect (VSD). □

109 Examination of a hypotonic, obese child reveals poorly developed gonads. □

110 A 4-year-old boy presents with moderate learning difficulties, characteristic facies – a long face and large, everted ears. Examination reveals large gonads. *fragile* ✗ □

111 A tall adolescent boy presents with gynaecomastia and poorly developed gonads. □

112 A child with a small lower jaw, a posteriorly displaced tongue and a midline cleft of the soft palate presents with feeding difficulties. □

---

113 A 62-year-old man presented with sudden-onset severe central chest pain, radiating between the shoulder blades. Which ONE of the following is true about acute aortic dissection?

A   Direct vasodilators eg sodium nitroprusside and diazoxide are the agents of choice for the control of blood pressure

B   Intravenous β-blockers are the agents of choice

C   Patients do not need to be on long-term antihypertensives after the dissection has been corrected

D   Surgery is the treatment of choice for uncomplicated and stable distal dissection

E   The 10-year survival rate for treated dissection is only 10%   □

---

114 A 4-week-old baby is diagnosed with congenital hypertrophic pyloric stenosis. Which ONE of the following is the best surgical procedure for this condition?

A   Belsey Mark IV operation   D   Pyloroplasty
B   Billroth I   E   Ramstedt's operation
C   Billroth II   *Pyloromyotomy*   □

Theme: **Investigation of endocrine disorders**

Options

A   Corticotrophin-releasing test
B   Dexamethasone suppression test
C   Glucose tolerance test
D   High/normal urine osmolality with low serum osmolality
E   Hypertension with hyperkalaemia
F   Hyponatraemia, hyperkalaemia, increased urea
G   Increased MIBG uptake
H   Increased serum 17-hydroxyprogesterone
I   Insulin-hypoglycaemia test
J   Low urine osmolality and higher serum osmolality
K   Short Synacthen® test

Instructions

For each of the patients described below choose the SINGLE most appropriate test or investigation finding from the list of options above. Each option may be used once, more than once or not at all.

115 A 46-year-old man presented with persistent frontal headache and visual disturbance. He was found to be hypertensive. He complained of tightening of his wedding ring and comparison with previous photographs shows a change in appearance. Which of the above tests will be diagnostic for this condition?

116 A 49-year-old man with a previous diagnosis of treated tuberculosis presented to his GP with tiredness, weakness and lethargy. The GP found oral pigmentation and postural hypotension. What is the initial diagnostic test in this case?

117 A 36-year-old woman with central weight gain, thin skin, oligomenorrhoea, and who was prone to easy bruising was also found to have impaired glucose tolerance. What is the most valuable test you could organise to diagnose this condition?

118 A 62-year-old man with known lung cancer presented with fits. He was found to have profound hyponatraemia. Which test result will point towards the diagnosis?

119 A mother brings her 15-year-old daughter to the GP complaining of severe acne and greasy skin. The girl also informs you that she has recently noticed an increase in facial hair. While taking the history you gather that she has not yet started to menstruate.   ☐

---

120 A 35-year-old lady comes to her GP complaining of heavy, painful periods. She gives a history of regular periods that have recently become heavy and painful, especially during the first 2 days. Physical examination is unremarkable. Which is the SINGLE most effective treatment for her condition?

A   Cyclical progesterone   D   Mefenamic acid and tranexamic acid
B   Endometrial ablation   E   Mirena® coil
C   Hysterectomy   ☐

---

121 A 66-year-old man presented with stridor and hoarseness of his voice. What is the best lung function variable to assist diagnosis of upper airway obstruction?

A   Flow volume loop   D   Spirometry
B   Mouth pressures   E   Transfer factor
C   Slow vital capacity measurement   ☐

---

122 A 36-year-old lady presented with haemoptysis and flitting pulmonary opacities. There was a long history of sinusitis. She then developed hypertension, proteinuria and peripheral oedema. Renal biopsy showed glomeruli containing areas fibrinoid necrosis and crescents in Bowman's space. What is the SINGLE most likely form of glomerular disease in this patient?

A   Diffuse proliferative glomerulonephritis
B   Focal segmental glomerulosclerosis
C   Membranoproliferative glomerulonephritis
D   Mesangial proliferative glomerulonephritis
E   Rapidly proliferative glomerulonephritis   ☐

Theme: **Diagnosis of mental illness**

Options

A	Abnormal bereavement reaction	G	Mood disorder secondary to alcohol misuse
B	Adjustment disorder		
C	Agoraphobia	H	Obsessive-compulsive disorder
D	Depression	I	Panic attack
E	Generalised anxiety state	J	Post-traumatic stress disorder
F	Mixed anxiety and depression	K	Social phobia

Instructions

For each of the patients described below choose the SINGLE most appropriate diagnosis from the list of options above. Each option may be used once, more than once or not at all.

123 A 37-year-old man has difficulty going to the supermarket and travelling away from home. ☐

124 A 32-year-old man appears a bit numb and anxious and is unable to drive since an accident 3 months ago. ☐

125 A 32-year-old woman has been feeling very apprehensive and tense in most situations and on most days over the last 7 months. ☐

126 A 67-year-old woman has kept her husband's room as it was before his death 2 years ago and no longer goes out to bingo as she used to. She often 'sees' her husband and says he is calling her to join him. ☐

127 A 23-year-old man often has thoughts that he might be harming children. He finds such thoughts hard to resist and, because of them, feels anxious, guilty and ashamed. ☐

128 A 22-year-old man has been diagnosed with testicular cancer. Which is the SINGLE most appropriate incision to make in order to perform a retroperitoneal lymph node dissection?

A	Grid-iron	D	Midline
B	Inguinal	E	Vertical scrotal
C	Lanz		

☐

Theme: **Causes of ascites**

Options

A	Budd–Chiari syndrome	F	Malignant ascites
B	Chronic pancreatitis	G	Meigs' syndrome
C	Chylous ascites	H	Nephrotic syndrome
D	Congestive cardiac failure	I	Tuberculous peritonitis
E	Constrictive pericarditis		

Instructions

For each of the patients described below choose the SINGLE most appropriate diagnosis from the list of options above. Each option may be used once, more than once or not at all.

129 A 46-year-old man went to his GP complaining of progressive swelling of the ankles and worsening ascites. Examination of the JVP showed a <u>prominent *y* descent.</u> ☐

130 A 48-year-old lady with known polycythaemia vera developed sudden-onset ascites, which was tender. ☐

131 A 43-year-old lady presented with fatigue, generalised lethargy, increasing abdominal girth and breathlessness. She was also amenorrhoeic. The CA-125 level was raised. ☐

132 A 36-year-old man who was undergoing treatment for lymphoma developed ascites. Examination of the fluid showed a raised triglyceride level. ☐

133 A 38-year-old man, known to be HIV-positive, comes to the hospital with breathlessness and increasing swelling of his abdomen. On examination, he is found to have moderate ascites. Straw-coloured fluid is drained from his abdomen and sent for examination. ☐

---

134 A 26-year-old lady comes to the gynaecology clinic with a history of recurrent second-trimester miscarriages. Which is the SINGLE most important factor that could explain this?

A	Antiphospholipid syndrome	D	Congenital toxoplasmosis
B	Cervical incompetence	E	Polycystic ovarian syndrome
C	Chromosomal abnormality		

☐

135 A 26-year-old medical house officer who had previously been vaccinated for hepatitis B was screened for immune status. Which ONE of the following patterns of serological results is consistent with hepatitis B immunity?

A   HbsAg-negative, anti HBs-negative, anti-HBc-negative, anti-Hbe-negative

B   HbsAg-negative, anti-HBs-negative, anti-HBc-negative, anti-Hbe-positive

C   HbsAg-negative, anti-HBs-positive, anti-HBc-negative, anti-Hbe-negative

D   HbsAg-negative, anti-HBs-positive, anti-HBc-positive, anti-Hbe-positive

E   HbsAg-positive, anti-HBs-positive, anti-HBc-positive, anti-Hbe-positive   ☐

Theme: **Joint pain and swelling**

Options

A   Ankylosing spondylitis
B   DLE
C   Golfer's elbow
D   Gout
E   Osgood–Schlatter disease
F   Osteoarthritis
G   Pseudogout
H   Psoriatic arthritis
I   Rheumatoid arthritis
J   SLE
K   Tennis elbow

Instructions

For each of the patients described below choose the SINGLE most appropriate diagnosis from the list of options above. Each option may be used once, more than once or not at all.

136 A 50-year-old man comes to A&E with a red, hot, and acutely tender right great toe. His uric acid level is normal.   ☐

137 A 34-year-old woman develops joint pain and swelling of the small joints of her hand, which has been progressive over the last 2years. X-rays of the affected joints show narrowing of joint spaces, osteoporosis and marginal erosions of the articulating bones.   ☐

138 A 47-year-old man complains of right elbow pain which developed after he painted his house over the weekend. Examination reveals tenderness over the lateral epicondyle. ☐

139 A 45-year-old woman presents with swelling of the DIP joints in both her hands. She has red scaly patches on her elbows. ☐

140 A 78-year-old woman presents with difficulty walking and pain over the last few months, which has made her more dependent on her Zimmer frame. She is upset that she can no longer do her shopping. ☐

---

141 A 32-year-old woman with grand mal epilepsy, who was on phenytoin, went her GP for advice regarding pregnancy. Which ONE of the following is inappropriate advice regarding pregnancy and epilepsy?

A   It is currently recommended that pregnant women are maintained on effective drug therapy during pregnancy

B   The mother should be treated with oral vitamin K in the last 2 weeks of pregnancy

C   The overall incidence of fetal abnormalities in children born to mothers with epilepsy is about 5-6%

D   The seizure frequency would be most likely to increase during pregnancy

E   When possible, it is prudent to put the patient on monotherapy at the lowest possible therapeutic dose, especially in the first trimester of pregnancy ☐

---

142 A 42-year-old woman has just returned from theatre after a thyroidectomy. What is the SINGLE most important investigation to perform after this operation?

A   ECG
B   Serum calcium
C   Serum magnesium

D   Serum potassium
E   Serum urea ☐

---

143 A 52-year-old man with a background history of type 2 diabetes, depression and Crohn's disease, developed progressive enlargement of a tarsometatarsal joint. The joint became progressively unstable, subluxed, and crepitus could be felt. Notably, he did not experience much pain. What is the most likely diagnosis?

A   Arthritis related to inflammatory bowel disease
B   Hypertrophic pulmonary osteoarthritis
C   Neuropathic joint disease
D   Psoriatic arthritis
E   Reactive arthritis

Theme: **Mineral deficiencies**

Options

A   Chromium deficiency   F   Manganese deficiency
B   Cobalt deficiency   G   Molybdenum deficiency
C   Copper deficiency   H   Phosphate deficiency
D   Fluoride deficiency   I   Selenium deficiency
E   Iodine deficiency   J   Zinc deficiency

Instructions

For each of the patients described below choose the SINGLE most likely mineral deficiency from the list of options above. Each option may be used once, more than once or not at all.

144 A 25-year-old man was diagnosed with diabetes and atherosclerosis. Which mineral deficiency may be the cause?

145 A 46-year-old man was found to have ischaemic heart disease and cardiomyopathy. He was also found to be infertile due to a reduced sperm count. His IgG and IgA levels were reduced. Which mineral deficiency may be responsible?

146 An 18-year-old man from the Middle East was found to have lack of sexual maturation, lack of pubic hair, and small stature. He also had a rash and diarrhoea. The rash was on the face, groin, hands and feet.

147 A patient on long-term total parenteral nutrition (TPN) developed a syndrome characterised by hypouricaemia, hypermethioninaemia, low urinary sulphate excretion, tachycardia, tachypnoea and mental and visual disturbances. ☐

148 A Highlander brings her child to the GP due to delayed growth spurt. While talking to the mother you gather that the child has also been a poor performer at school. ☐

---

149 A 9-year-old girl attends the rheumatology outpatient department for investigation of chronic joint pains which are predominantly affecting her left hip, right knee and left shoulder. Which ONE of the following statements regarding juvenile chronic arthritis (JCA) is correct?

A   Antinuclear antibody test is usually negative

B   Corticosteroids are the most appropriate treatment for acute exacerbations

C   Lymphadenitis makes an alternative diagnosis more likely

D   Regular slit-lamp examination should be performed

E   Rheumatoid factor is usually positive ☐

---

150 A 4-month-old previoulsy healthy baby boy was found dead in his cot. A thorough investigation and complete autopsy failed to reveal the cause of death. Which SINGLE factor is most associated with an increased incidence of such deaths in infants?

A   Breast-feeding

B   High socioeconomic class

C   Low parity

D   Warm summer months

E   Young maternal age ☐

Theme: **Poisoning**

Options

A   Arsenic
B   Aspirin
C   Cyanide
D   Digoxin
E   Iron

F   Lead
G   Lithium
H   Mercury
I   Methanol
J   Organophosphates

Instructions

For each of the patients described below choose the SINGLE most likely agent from the list of options above. Each option may be used once, more than once or not at all.

151 A 38-year-old farmer presented with profuse vomiting, lacrimation, blurring of vision and small pupils. The diagnosis was made by the measurement of blood acetylcholinesterase, which was less than 50% of normal. ☐

152 A 32-year-old lady presented with generalised muscle weakness, pronounced tremor, and choreoathetosis. The ECG showed ST depression and T-wave inversion. ☐

153 A 32-year-old man who works in the spraying industry presented with headaches, confusion and drowsiness. Other signs and symptoms included skin thickening, fluid accumulation (resulting in puffiness), especially around the lower eyelids, face and ankles, diarrhoea, garlic breath, perspiration, excessive salivation, generalised itching, oral inflammation, sore throat, runny nose, excessive tearing, numbness, skin inflammation, hair loss, weakness, and loss of appetite. The diagnosis was made by examination of his hair. ☐

154 An 18-year-old man presented with behavioural changes, avoiding social contact, and introverted behaviour. He then developed ataxia and involuntary muscle spasms. He also developed gum bleeding and a metallic taste in the mouth. ☐

155 An 18-year-old man working in a scrapyard presented with nausea and vomiting. He also complained of severe abdominal cramps. He has also recently noticed weakness in his right wrist and difficulty in lifting it. A routine blood test shows him to be anaemic. ☐

---

156 A 4-year-old child has swallowed a one-pence coin and an X-ray shows it to be at the level of the stomach. What is the SINGLE best management?

A   Endoscopy
B   Laparoscopy
C   Laparotomy

D   Leave alone
E   Tracheostomy

☐

---

157 A 64-year-old man with long-standing hypertension presents to his GP with a painful left first metatarsophalangeal joint, which is red and tender and associated with limited movement. A diagnosis of acute gout is made, and the patient is commenced on ibuprofen for pain relief. Which ONE of the following statements regarding acute gout is correct?

A   Allopurinol treatment should be initiated early to reduce the duration of symptoms
B   Colchicine gives effective pain relief but is frequently associated with profuse diarrhoea
C   Gout is more common in patients with contact dermatitis
D   Raised serum urate concentrations confirm the diagnosis
E   The risk of recurrent attacks decreases with advancing age ☐

---

158 During your examination of a newborn baby you fail to feel the testicles in the scrotum. You explain to his parents that he has undescended testes. Which SINGLE statement best fits with this condition?

A   10% of neonates have undescended testes at birth
B   Intranasal gonadotrophin-releasing hormone is the treatment of choice
C   Orchidopexy reduces the chances of later malignancy
D   Orchidopexy within 2years eliminates the chance of the child becoming infertile
E   'Undescended testis' is usually bilateral ☐

Theme: **Urogenital problems**

Options

A   Atrophic trigonitis

B   Cystocele

C   Detrusor overactivity (DO)

D   Genuine stress incontinence (GSI)

E   Interstitial cystitis

F   Procidentia

G   Pyelonephritis

H   Rectocele

I   Urinary tract infection

J   Vault prolapse

K   Vesico-vaginal fistula

Instructions

For each of the clinical scenarios described below choose the SINGLE most appropriate diagnosis from the list of options given above. Each option may be used once, more than once or not at all.

159 A 58-year-old woman comes to your clinic complaining of urinary incontinence. She says she wets herself before she has a chance to get to the toilet. The symptoms have recently become so bad that she has to wear incontinence pads all the time. She even finds it difficult to go out shopping as she feels like going to the toilet all the time. However, on going to the toilet she only passes very small amounts of urine. ☐

160 A 62-year-old woman comes to the gynaecological clinic complaining of urinary incontinence. She says that she wets herself when she coughs or sneezes but has no problems at other times. She has also recently noticed a 'lump' in her vagina which comes down on straining in the toilet. On examination, you notice that the womb is well supported but when you ask her to cough she becomes incontinent and there is moderate descent of the anterior vaginal wall. ☐

161 A 26-year-old woman comes to A&E complaining of passing clear, water-like discharge from her vagina. She says that it smells like urine and is quite embarrassing when she is having intercourse. She now has to wear sanitary towels all the time. While taking a history, you gather that she has recently given birth, when she had an instrumental delivery. ☐

162 An anxious 34-year-old woman comes to the clinic complaining of increased urinary frequency for the last 6months. She has been treated with many different antibiotics by her GP for repeated bouts of cystitis but there has been no improvement in her symptoms. All mid-stream urine cultures have been negative. ☐

163 While seeing an 85-year-old woman in a care home because of urinary retention, you notice a large lump coming out of the introitus. ☐

---

164 A 36-year-old woman is treated with multiple medications. Two months ago, she gave birth to a healthy baby girl. Which ONE of the following drugs, when given to a breast-feeding mother are regarded as potentially hazardous to a newborn child?

A Amiodarone   D Theophylline
B Aspirin   E Warfarin
C Paracetamol   ☐

---

165 You are asked to assess a 17-year-old girl with weight loss and dieting. You suspect her to be suffering from anorexia nervosa. Which SINGLE criterion gives a diagnosis of classic anorexia nervosa?

A 70% of expected weight for age and height
B 75% of expected weight for age and height
C 80% of expected weight for age and height
D 85% of expected weight for age and height
E 90% of expected weight for age and height   ☐

---

166 A 42-year-old woman is admitted to A&E with reduced conscious level. She is found to have shallow respirations, pinpoint pupils and a blood pressure of 88/64 mmHg. The ambulance crew report finding empty packets of tablets at the call scene. Which ONE of the following, taken in overdose, is most likely to account for these features?

A Amitriptyline   D Ecstasy
B Co-codamol   E Ibuprofen
C Diazepam   ☐

Theme: **Site of neurological lesions**

Options

A   Left frontal cortex

B   Left parietal region

C   Left temporoparietal region

D   Right frontal cortex

E   Right parietal region

F   Right temporal region

G   Occipital region

Instructions

For each of the patients described below choose the SINGLE most likely site of neurological involvement from the list of options above. Each option may be used once, more than once or not at all.

167 A 62-year-old man developed loss of fine movements and strength in the arms, hands and fingers on the right side. There was disinhibition of social and sexual behaviour. There was lack of control of language-related movement. ☐

168 A 48-year-old smoker developed inability to write or do arithmetic and lack of skilled movement. There was also confusion in trying to distinguish between right and left sides. ☐

169 A 72-year-old man developed difficulty in short-term memory and facial recognition. This was followed by anterograde amnesia. ☐

170 An 80-year-old blind man denied his visual impairment. The patient attempted to walk, bumping into objects and injuring himself. ☐

171 A 60-year-old man is referred to the psychiatric clinic because he has been confused and acting strangely recently. His relatives report that it has been difficult to understand what he has been saying lately as he speaks meaningless nonsense. ☐

rolled edge w/ central ulceration

172 A 76-year-old man presents with a lesion on the cheek, just above the junction of the angle of the mouth and tragus. The lesion has rolled-over edges. What is the SINGLE most likely diagnosis?

A   Basal cell carcinoma   D   Solar keratosis
B   Keratoachanthoma   E   Squamous cell carcinoma
C   Melanoma   ☐

Theme: **Head injury**

Options

A   Base of skull fracture   F   Le Fort I fracture
B   Concussion   G   Le Fort II fracture
C   *Contrecoup* injury   H   Le Fort III fracture
D   Extradural haemorrhage   I   Subarachnoid haemorrhage
E   Intracerebral haemorrhage   J   Subdural haemorrhage

Instructions

For each of the patients described below choose the SINGLE most appropriate diagnosis from the list of options above. Each option may be used once, more than once or not at all.

173 A 26-year-old man was in the street outside a pub when he was hit with a heavy object on the right side of his head. Now in the A&E resuscitation unit, his airway is clear and he is breathing spontaneously. His GCS score is 8. There is bruising over the left mastoid process.   ☐

174 A 17-year-old boy was brought into A&E after being hit on the side of his head by a cricket ball during a match. He fell to the ground immediately and was unresponsive for a few seconds, but then recovered completely. After a while it was noticed that his conscious level was deteriorating. His present GCS score is 7 and he has an ipsilateral dilated pupil.   ☐

175 A 63-year-old man presents to A&E very confused. He is known to be an alcoholic and has a history of recurrent falls.   ☐

176 A 4-year-old child fell from a swing and hit his head. He did not lose consciousness but vomited once. He says that only his head hurts. No neurological abnormalities can be found.   ☐

177 A 50-year-old man fell from a 3.6-m- (12-ft-) high ladder and hit the back of his head, after which he lost consciousness. He has been brought to A&E and has not regained consciousness. ☐

---

178 A 65-year-old man is rushed to the resuscitation room of the local A&E after a sudden collapse. He is unconscious, his blood pressure is recorded as 50/32 mmHg in his right arm, and a cardiac monitor shows a broad-complex tachycardia. Which ONE of the following is the most appropriate initial management?

A   DC cardioversion
B   Intravenous adenosine
C   Intravenous adrenaline (epinephrine)
D   Intravenous amiodarone
E   Intravenous metoprolol ☐

---

179 A 35-year-old lady comes to your gynaecology clinic with sudden onset of hirsutism. She also describes secondary amenorrhoea and baldness over the last 6months. Blood investigations reveal markedly raised levels of serum testosterone (almost ten times the normal level). Among other blood tests, FBC, U&Es and LFTs are normal. What is the SINGLE best diagnosis for the condition described above?

A   Anorexia nervosa
B   Menopause
C   Ovarian thecoma
D   Polycystic ovarian syndrome (PCOS)
E   Premature ovarian failure ☐

Theme: **Pyrexia of unknown origin**

Options

A	Brucellosis	F	Pancreatic carcinoma
B	EBV infection	G	Polyarteritis nodosa
C	Familial Mediterranean fever	H	Q fever Coxiella Burretil
D	Kawasaki disease	I	SLE
E	Lymphoma	J	Thyrotoxicosis

Instructions

For each of the patients described below choose the SINGLE most appropriate diagnosis from the list of options above. Each option may be used once, more than once or not at all.

180 A 36-year-old man of Arab descent developed fever with recurrent episodes of abdominal pain. He also suffered from pain in the ankles and hip. He also had skin lesions varying in diameter from 8 cm to 12 cm. Blood tests revealed a raised white cell count, ESR, serum haptoglobin and caeruloplasmin level. Treatment was with colchicine. ☐

181 A 5-year-old girl developed high fever with conjunctivitis. A few days later a rash appeared over the trunk and genital area. The palms of her hands and the soles of her feet started to look swollen, purplish-red, and irritated. ☐

182 A 26-year-old man developed high fevers, severe headache, general malaise, myalgia, confusion, sore throat, chills, sweats and a non-productive cough. He also had nausea, vomiting, diarrhoea, abdominal pain and chest pain. The fever usually lasted for 1 week. He lost some weight. He also developed pneumonia, with altered liver function tests. The diagnosis was clinched by the indirect immunofluorescence test. ☐

183 A 45-year-old lady presented with acute abdominal pain, haematuria and proteinuria. There was a purpuric rash all over the body. Angiography demonstrated microaneuryms in the hepatic, intestinal and renal vessels. ☐

184 A 22-year-old woman presents with fever, sore throat and feeling very weak. She also complains of severe chest pain. On examination you find generalised lymphadenopathy with hepatosplenomegaly. ☐

185 A 22-year-old woman burned the palm of her right hand while trying to take the lid off a pan while she was cooking. Which ONE of the following is the most likely percentage of burn she has suffered?

A   1% burn

B   5% burn

C   10% burn

D   20% burn

E   30% burn

186 A 78-year-old woman is found collapsed at home by a neighbour, and brought to A&E. She has reduced conscious level, with signs of a flaccid left hemiparesis. She appears dehydrated, has a blood pressure of 94/60 mmHg, and there is some bruising overlying the right buttock and thigh. Initial investigations show: sodium 138mmol/l, potassium 4.6 mmol/l, urate 0.82 mmol/l, urea 31 mmol/l, creatinine 486 µmol/l and creatine kinase (CK) 185,000 U/l. Which ONE of the following would be the most appropriate early treatment?

A   Intravenous 5% dextrose at 125 ml/h

B   Intravenous 1.26% sodium bicarbonate at 250 ml/h

C   Intravenous streptokinase

D   Rectal aspirin 300 mg

E   Urgent haemodialysis

Theme: **Anaemia in children**

Options

A   Aplastic anaemia

B   G6PD deficiency

C   Hereditary spherocytosis

D   Iron deficiency anaemia

E   Pyruvate kinase deficiency

F   Sickle cell disease

G   Thalassaemia

Instructions

For each of the patients described below choose the SINGLE most appropriate diagnosis from the list of options above. Each option may be used once, more than once or not at all.

187 A 9-month-old Afro-Caribbean child presents with painful swelling in her fingers and toes and with mild anaemia.

188 A 3-year-old child attends with jaundice and anaemia, failure to thrive and maxillary overgrowth. ☐

189 A child of Mediterranean origin presents with jaundice, pallor and dark urine, following a course of ciprofloxacin. ☐

190 A 2-year-old child, who is a very fussy eater, has started to eat soil while playing in the garden. ☐

---

191 A 73-year-old man with dementia is brought to A&E by his wife. She states that over the past 24 hours he has inadvertently taken around 22 of her 500-mg paracetamol tablets (11 g). He is asymptomatic, and cannot recall taking any tablets. He appears well nourished (weight 70 kg), and clinical examination is normal. Which ONE of the following would be appropriate?

A   Check LFTs and, if normal, discharge home from A&E
B   Check LFTs and prothrombin time and, if normal, discharge home from A&E
C   If serum paracetamol is below the 4-hour treatment level, take no further action
D   Monitor clinical signs for 24 hours and discharge home if he remains well
E   N-acetylcysteine infusion should be commenced and LFTs checked at 24 hours ☐

---

192 An 11-year-old boy has been observed not to enjoy contact sports, likes dressing like a girl and is keen to imitate effeminate stereotypes. He has had an otherwise normal development. This behaviour is persistent over time and he is now referred following bullying in school. What is the SINGLE most likely cause in this case?

A   Congenital adrenal hyperplasia   D   Klinefelter's syndrome
B   Fetishism   E   Transvestism
C   Gender identity disorder   ☐

Theme: **Treatment of hypertension**

Options

A	Amlodipine	F	Moxonidine
B	Atenolol	G	Perindopril
C	Bendroflumethiazide	H	Prazosin
D	Doxazosin	I	Sodium nitroprusside
E	Losartan	J	Verapamil

Instructions

For each of the patients described below choose the SINGLE most appropriate drug treatment from the list of options above. Each option may be used once, more than once or not at all.

193 A 56-year-old man had an MI. According to the EUROPA study, the prescription of which agent will significantly reduce the incidence of recurrent MI? ☐

194 A 58-year-old man had an MI. The prescription of which agent within 12 hours will reduce the extension of the infarct? ☐

195 A 57-year-old man was going for surgery on his aortic aneurysm. What would the agent of choice for induction of controlled hypotension be? ☐

196 A 42-year-old man was diagnosed with mild hypertension that required treatment. He was also obese and had insulin-resistant diabetes. The prescription of which antihypertensive agent would also improve insulin sensitivity? ☐

197 A 45-year-old man, diagnosed with hypertension, was started on ACE inhibitors by his GP. Unfortunately, he soon developed intractable cough and had to discontinue the treatment. What is the best alternative antihypertensive drug for this patient, considering the side-effect described? ☐

198 A 26-year-old woman and her 28-year-old partner come to the
GP surgery complaining of primary infertility for 2 years. She
gives a history of irregular menstrual cycles. What is the SINGLE
best test to see whether she is ovulating or not?

A   Basal body temperature estimation
B   Cervical fern test
C   Day 2 LH and FSH
D   Day 21 progesterone level
E   Endometrial biopsy
□

199 You are asked to review the medications of an elderly patient
admitted for assessment of recurrent falls. Which ONE of the
following drugs should be used with particular caution in elderly
patients?

A   Bumetanide   D   Paracetamol
B   Metronidazole   E   Phenytoin
C   Omeprazole
□

200 You are planning to perform a circumcision on a 25-year-old man
with a history of balanitis xerotica obliterans as a day case procedure.
He has no other medical problems. What is the American Society of
Anesthesiologists *(ASA) classification for this surgery?*

A   ASA 1   D   ASA 4
B   ASA 2   E   ASA 5
C   ASA 3
□

Practice Paper – Answers

1   C: Haemochromatosis
Autosomal recessive inherited disorder of iron metabolism,
characterised by excessive accumulation of iron in various organs.
This results in clinical symptoms of hepatic failure, diabetes
mellitus, cardiomyopathy, gonadal failure and arthropathy.

2   A: α_1-Antitrypsin deficiency
Once again, an autosomal dominant inherited disorder, which is
very prevalent in Northern Europe. Alpha$_1$-antitrypsin, which is a
glycoprotein, is one of the protein inhibitors responsible for
various inflammatory responses. As a result of its decreased
synthesis there are clinical manifestations in the form of
emphysema (specially among smokers) and liver disease.

3   J: Wilson's disease
This disease is also known as 'hepatolenticular degeneration'. It is
a rare autosomal recessively inherited disorder of copper
metabolism, characterised by increased deposits of copper in
various organs, mainly in the liver and basal ganglia of the brain.
The neurological symptoms are due to the degenerative changes
in the basal ganglia.

4   G: Lupoid hepatitis
Also known as chronic autoimmune hepatitis (CAH). Mainly
seen in women, the condition is most likely to be caused by
immunological disturbances. Other autoimmune conditions
often co-exist. There is hypergammaglobulinaemia and
antinuclear, anti-smooth muscle and anti-liver/kidney
microsomal antibodies in the serum. Treatment involves
long-term steroid and immunosupressive therapy.

5   H: Primary biliary cirrhosis (PBC)
This chronic liver disease is characterised by progressive
destruction of the bile ducts, resulting in cirrhosis. It is also
known as 'chronic non-suppurative destructive cholangitis',
thereby emphasising the fact that cirrhosis is only a late feature of

the disease. It is mainly seen among women and pruritus is the dominant feature during the early stages of the disease. The aetiology is most probably related to damaged cell-mediated immunity. This condition is also associated with other autoimmune disorders.

---

6   D: Platelet count 60 × 10⁹/l

'HELLP' stands for 'haemolysis, elevated liver enzymes and low platelets'. Although an extremely rare occurrence in pregnancy (incidence of 0.1–0.6%), in pre-eclampsia this rate increases to 4–12%. This is associated with raised blood pressure and microangiopathic haemolytic anaemia. The symptoms are those of jaundice, secondary to the haemolysis, which results in the blood picture of a low haemoglobin and a raised bilirubin. The patient also complains of epigastric pain due to the stretching of the liver capsule. There is also derangement of the liver functions due to excessive haemolysis, resulting in the elevated liver enzymes. The management involves supportive treatment to the mother and prompt delivery of the fetus.

---

7   C: Heparin is added to the solution

Sepsis related to urinary catheters is most commonly due to Gram-negative bacilli or anaerobic organisms. Heparin is usually added to TPN solution to reduce the risk of central venous access-related thrombosis, which is more likely during TPN infusion than during administration of crystalloid solutions because of local vascular inflammation. Electrolytes should be checked daily after commencing TPN, and the content of potassium, magnesium, calcium and other elements in the solution can be varied to maintain homeostasis. Nitrogen balance, determined by urea, albumin and total protein, is less critical and can be measured weekly. Acute hyperglycaemia and hyperlipidaemia are recognised consequences of TPN feeding, particularly in patients with diabetes mellitus. Blood glucose should therefore be monitored carefully when TPN is started.

---

8   A: Aortic rupture

Chest X-rays are performed as part of the protocol of the Advanced Trauma Life Support (ATLS) guidelines. A patient in shock with a widened mediastinum points to the fact that the mediastinum is filling up with blood from the great vessels, something that occurs in high-energy impact accidents.

9   D: Intracranial bleeding

Any impact to the head combined with a focal neurological deficit would point towards a very serious injury and requires immediate action.

10   H: Tension pneumothorax

In this case the pneumothorax could have developed as a result of anaesthetic intervention or, alternatively, the patient could have a concomitant chest injury that was dormant at the time of presentation.

11   E: Ruptured bronchus

If there is no improvement in symptoms following insertion of a chest drain, there must be some other pathological condition present. In this case the pneumomediastinum provides the clue.

12   C: Flail chest

When a segment of a rib is fractured it becomes separated and moves independently (the 'flail segment').

---

13   A: 20% of people who regularly drink develop cirrhosis of liver

Autopsy reports indicate a high prevalence of cirrhosis in regular drinkers, and the likelihood increases with the duration of the heavy drinking pattern. The clinical incidence of complications due to cirrhosis is somewhat lower. The risk of cirrhosis is greatest in those with a regular drinking pattern, for example daily consumption. An intermittent 'binge drinking' pattern less commonly causes cirrhosis than the same overall alcohol intake during regular drinking. However, binge drinking is associated with a higher incidence of cardiomyopathy, acute pancreatitis, and accidental injury. Pregnant women should be advised to abstain from alcohol for the duration of pregnancy to minimise the risks of fetal alcohol syndrome and subsequent developmental delay in the newborn. Short-term adverse effects, including headache and nausea during 'hangover', are often caused by congeners such as isomayl alcohol or metabolites such as acetaldehyde, rather than being a direct toxic effect of alcohol itself.

14 E: Vitamin D-resistant rickets

Colour blindness and haemophilia are X-linked recessive disorders. Achondroplasia is an autosomal dominant condition and phenylketonuria is an autosomal recessive disorder. Vitamin D-resistant rickets is an X-linked dominant disorder. It is a rare condition which can affect either sex.

15 C: Guttate psoriasis

The lesion described is classically seen in psoriasis, commonly over the extensor surfaces of the elbows and knees and in the scalp. Infection is considered to be an aggravating factor.

16 H: Porphyria cutanea tarda

This is also known as 'cutaneous hepatic porphyria' or 'cutaneous, non-acute manifestation of hepatic porphyria'. The diagnosis depends on the increased levels of uroporphyrin in the urine. There is perivascular deposition of periodic acid-Schiff (PAS) stain in the blisters. Venesection and chloroquine may play a role in the remission phase.

① bullous reacn to sunlight
② hyperpigmentation + scarring
③ liver dse

17 B: Dermatitis herpetiformis

This is commonly seen in patients with gluten-sensitive enteropathy. One of the main features of this lesion is that it is extremely itchy. This condition is treated with dapsone, which controls the rash within hours.

18 D: Lichen planus

Chloroquine is the obvious aggravating factor here. Treatment in this acute-phase eruption usually involves topical corticosteriod and antihistamines.

19 I: Seborrhoeic dermatitis

This is usually seen in areas that have more sebaceous glands. The scalp is the principal area involved among other areas, such as the eyebrows, nasolabial folds, the ears and the neck. There may be associated bacterial infection resulting in folliculitis and abscess formation.

---

20 E: Salvage cystectomy
The patient has already been treated with radiotherapy and chemotherapy and as the tumour is extensive but still contained within the bladder walls it is best to perform a salvage cystectomy to prevent further spread, avoid urinary obstruction and prolong survival.

---

21 A: In severe ulcerative colitis, patients who do not respond to high-dose intravenous steroids may respond to azathioprine
Mild attacks of ulcerative colitis may respond to local administration of corticosteroid treatment. However, moderate or severe ulcerative colitis relapse usually requires systemic administration of high-dose corticosteroids, and rectal administration alone is inadequate. Severe attacks of ulcerative colitis are associated with a high mortality rate (up to 10%). Azathioprine increases the remission rate for severe relapses when used in addition to systemic corticosteroid treatment, or in patients who have failed to respond to corticosteroids alone. Sulfasalazine is ineffective in the treatment of an acute relapse, but is a useful maintenance treatment for long-term prevention of ulcerative colitis attacks. Discontinuation of sulfasalazine is associated with a high relapse rate, and many patients benefit from lifelong treatment.

---

22 H: Herpes hominis
Neonatal herpes infection is commonly due to herpes simplex type 2 virus. Active herpetic lesions anywhere in the birth canal is an indication for elective Caesarean section. There is about a 40% risk of direct infection during the infant's passage through the birth canal. Neonatal herpes usually manifests in the first 3 weeks after birth with localised skin lesions in the form of vesicular and

pustular blisters. The virus can be isolated from the fluid taken from the blister. The presence of generalised viraemia results in systemic manifestations like jaundice, encephalopathy, petechiae and seizures. Neonatal HSV infection should be treated with intravenous aciclovir.

23   D: Congenital toxoplasmosis

Toxoplasma gondii, a protozoan parasite, is responsible for this disease. Infection occurs by eating undercooked meat. Only in 10% of women affected by the infection in the first trimester of pregnancy, does the infection result in clinical features in the baby. The diagnosis is made on the basis of rising antibody titres. Treatment with spiramycin may reduce the risk of transmission of infection to the fetus. Mental handicap and other neurological abnormalities manifest later in life.

24   J: Listeriosis

Maternal infection caused by the Gram-positive bacteria, *Listeria monocytogenes* may result in premature labour, stillbirth, recurrent miscarriages or fetal infection. Although a rare infection now, it was very prevalent not long ago. It is acquired by drinking unpasteurised milk and by eating other milk products such as cheese. It typically presents with vague flu-like symptoms and is usually treated with intravenous ampicillin and gentamicin during the acute phase.

25   I: HIV

Approximately a third of babies born to HIV-infected mothers will be affected. This figure is higher in underdeveloped countries where antiretroviral prophylaxis during labour is not available. The rate of disease progression in the affected group depends upon several factors like early detection and treatment, nutrition and host immunity. Many of the undiagnosed children may present initially with failure to thrive and repeated opportunistic infections.

26   C: Congenital syphilis

Congenital syphilis is a rare entity nowadays with the introduction of antenatal screening. The clinical signs described are classically found in syphilitic patients. 'Snuffle' is described as nasal discharge with infection, which is found in the early stages of congenital syphilis. Hutchinson's teeth are seen in the later stages of the disease.

---

27   B: Pallor and unresponsiveness during the collapse, followed by facial flushing and rapid recovery suggest transient bradyarrhythmia as a cause

Collapse associated with transient unconsciousness is typically due to an underlying cardiac cause or seizure. Short-lived limb twitching is a non-specific sign that is not diagnostic of epilepsy, and is often observed in the setting of cerebral hypoperfusion. Cardiac causes of collapse include myocardial infarction and arrhythmia. Transient bradyarrhythmia and vasovagal syncope are often associated with pallor and sweating, followed by a rapid recovery of full conscious level. A raised D-dimer test, even in the context of high clinical suspicion, does not establish the diagnosis of thromboembolic disease, and more detailed investigation is required (eg lung perfusion scan or CT pulmonary angiography). A normal D-dimer test, in the setting of low clinical suspicion, can be used to exclude the diagnosis in certain situations, however. Addisonian crises are characteristically associated with hypotension, hypoglycaemia and hyperkalaemia. Syncope is an uncommon feature of severe thyrotoxicosis, and an alternative cause should be sought.

---

28   D: Inform the DVLA

This is a non-discretionary requirement by law. It is good practice to discuss your course of action with his family and also to inform him before contacting the DVLA, but this is discretionary. It is the duty of anybody who is driving and/or holds a valid driving licence to inform the DVLA of any new or worsening medical condition. It is also the duty of the prescriber to inform the patient of the effect of his condition and of the medication prescribed on his 'fitness to drive'.

---

29   H: *Toxoplasma gondii* chorioretinitis

Toxoplasma gondii commonly causes cerebral abscesses and encephalitis as manifestations of cerebral toxoplasmosis in the AIDS patient.

30   B: CMV retinitis
This is the commonest cause of eye disease in these patients. 'Pizza eye appearance' is due to the haemorrhages and exudates seen in the retina. Floaters, scotomas, orbital pain and loss of visual acuity are some of the other features of CMV retinitis.

31   C: Kaposi's sarcoma of the conjunctiva
This is characterised by proliferation of vascular endothelial cells and may manifest locally (the most common cutaneous manifestation) or systemically. Local manifestations generally respond well to radiotherapy.

32   D: Orbital lymphoma
Primary non-Hodgkin's lymphoma in the CNS is usually seen in the later stages of the disease and patients respond poorly to treatment. However, if it is outside the CNS, these tumours usually manifest at an earlier stage and have a better prognosis.

33   G: Syphilitic anterior and posterior uveitis
This is a rare manifestation which is seen in the later stages of the disease. A red and painful eye is seen in anterior uveitis while progressive loss of vision is a feature of posterior uveitis. Syphilitic hepatitis is a poor prognostic factor.

---

34   E: Prilocaine
Bupivacaine should not be used for a Bier's block as it is cardiotoxic.

---

35   D: Pulsus bisferiens
The clinical features strongly suggest hypertrophic cardiomyopathy (HCMP). This condition often manifests as a sudden unexplained collapse, or as a sudden cardiac death. The mechanism of collapse can be arrhythmia (as suggested by the clinical scenario) or aortic outflow tract obstruction. Arrhythmias arise in this condition due to the disorganised myocardial architecture and abnormal conduction. Pulsus bisferiens is a rare clinical sign that is pathognomonic of HCMP with obstructed aortic outflow, and is characterised by a staggered, jerky pulse character. Obstruction occurs because of septal hypertrophy

encroaching into the aortic outflow tract, and due to disordered myocardial contractility.

---

36   B: Erythema infectiosum

Erythema infectiosum (also known as 'fifth disease') is caused by parvovirus B19 infection. It is a common disease in the spring months. The disease is transmitted by respiratory secretion, by vertical transmission from the mother to the fetus and by the transfusion of contaminated blood products. It starts with a fever, headache and myalgia, followed by a characteristic rash over the cheeks one week later. An aplastic crisis may occur in children with chronic haemolytic anaemia due to parvovirus infection and this is the most serious complication of parvovirus infection. Maternal parvovirus infection may lead to fetal hydrops.

37   E: Kawasaki disease

Kawasaki disease affects children between the ages of 6 months and 4 years. It affects the coronary arteries in about a third of children within the first 6 weeks of illness, and can cause myocardial ischaemia and death. The mortality rate is 1–2%. Clinical features include a fever of more than 5 days' duration, together with four out of five of the following features:

- conjunctival infection
- mucous membrane changes (dry lips, strawberry tongue)
- cervical lymphadenopathy
- rash
- red and oedematous palms and soles, followed by skin peeling.

38   I: Rubella

Rubella is generally a mild disease in children. Common in the spring and winter months, it is transmitted by the respiratory route. The prodrome is mild, with a low-grade fever. A maculopapular rash starts on the face and spreads centrifugally, then fades in 3–5 days. Lymphadenopathy, particularly of the suboccipital and postauricular nodes, is prominent. Complications are rare in children but include arthritis, encephalitis, thrombocytopenia and myocarditis.

39 A: Chickenpox

Chickenpox is caused by the varicella zoster virus and is spread by the respiratory route. Rashes come in crops for 3–5 days, and consist of papules, vesicles, pustules and crusts. Complications include meningitis, encephalitis and pneumonia.

40 G: Meningococcal meningitis

Any febrile child with a purpuric rash should be assumed to have meningococcal sepsis. Infants may present with poor feeding, irritability, drowsiness, seizures and reduced consciousness. Bulging fontanelle, neck stiffness and opisthotonos are late features.

41 C: Lithium

Chronic lithium treatment, even within the normal therapeutic range, causes a post-receptor defect of both TSH and ADH receptors. The former causes primary hypothyroidism, while the latter causes diabetes insipidus. Circulating ADH concentrations are normal, and administration of ADH (vasopressin) is unlikely to be of benefit due to end-organ insensitivity. Activity of TSH and ADH receptors can be restored after discontinuation of lithium, but this takes several days to weeks and function may not completely recover.

42 D: Moclobemide

All the other options reduce seizure threshold and therefore increase the risk of precipitating seizures.

43 E: Pulmonary infarction

This is secondary to migration of tumour cells.

44 D: Mesothelioma

This is a lung tumour arising from the pleura. There may be a history of exposure to asbestos, mainly the crocidolite (blue asbestos) variety. Progressive dyspnoea and pleuritic pain are the principal symptoms. There may be unilateral or bilateral pleural effusion.

45 H: SLE

This is a multi-organ, autoimmune, connective tissue disorder characterised by generalised vasculitis and the presence of antinuclear antibodies in almost all cases. The lung manifestations include pleural effusion, pleurisy, pneumonia and restrictive lung disease.

46 A: Hypothyroidism

The clue lies in the classic symptoms that have been described in the clinical scenario. Pleural effusion in hypothyroidism is due to an increase in ADH secretion and impaired water clearance, resulting in an electrolyte imbalance.

47 I: Tuberculosis

Tuberculosis is once again on the rise in the UK, mainly among the immigrant population. Although the X-ray findings alone suggest tuberculosis, every effort should be made to obtain microbiological evidence to help in the treatment. Sputum staining for AAFB (alcohol/acid-fast bacilli) using a ZN stain, sputum culture, fibreoptic bronchoscopy, and biopsies from pleura, lymph nodes and other lesions form the mainstay of diagnosis.

---

48 D: 1 in 380

The association of the risk of Down's syndrome with maternal age is:

All ages 1 in 650	37 years 1 in 240
30 years 1 in 900	40 years 1 in 110
35 years 1 in 380	44 years 1 in 37

---

49 C: Medullary carcinoma of the thyroid

Medullary carcinoma of the thyroid is often functional, associated with overproduction of calcitonin, and hypercalcaemia is a recognised feature. Medullary carcinoma can occur in the setting of multiple endocrine neoplasia, including phaeochromocytoma, Cushing's syndrome and parathyroid hyperplasia (MEN type 2A). In type 2B MEN, patients can have a marfanoid phenotype, and can have multiple ganglioneuromas affecting viscera, intestine and mucous membranes. Medullary thyroid carcinoma should be treated by surgical resection, and additional endocrine disorders sought. Consideration should be given to screening family members for occult endocrine disease.

---

50 A: Austin Moore hemiarthroplasty
In this case there is a high chance of avascular necrosis of the femoral head and a prosthesis (Austin Moore) is the solution.

51 D: Dynamic hip screw
Dynamic hip screws are used for intertrochanteric fractures.

52 B: Cannulated screws
As this is a relatively young patient, there is a chance to save the femoral head.

53 I: Thomas splint
In the setting of an A&E department, a Thomas splint is used as the initial management for hip and thigh injuries.

54 C: Distal condylar screws
Distal condylar screws are used in cases of infratrochanteric femoral fracture.

---

55 C: Normal-pressure hydrocephalus
Normal-pressure hydrocephalus is associated with expanded cerebral ventricles without significant cortical atrophy. Characteristic features are dementia, ataxia and urinary incontinence. A number of important clinical conditions can cause dementia and, in elderly patients, depression can be associated with memory impairment and slowed cognition and can be mistaken for early dementia. Depression would not be expected to cause ataxia or incontinence, however. Huntington's disease is an autosomal dominant disease that is typically associated with progressive chorea and dementia, and the movement disorder is often the prominent feature. Parkinson's disease typically manifests as resting tremor, rigidity and akinesia, and patients often come to medical attention due to falls and postural instability. Thiamine deficiency is usually associated with chronic alcohol excess, and causes cardiomyopathy,

polyneuropathy and amnesia. Wernicke–Korsakoff syndrome is associated with severe thiamine deficiency and typical features include nystagmus, ataxia and confusion. If suspected, the patient should be treated urgently with high doses of thiamine.

---

56   C: *BRCA1*

Around 25% of women with breast cancer have some family history of the disease but only 5–10% of these women show specific DNA changes related to the inherited gene. The risk factors associated with inheriting the oncogenes *BRCA1* or *BRCA2* are:

- family history of two or more relatives with breast or ovarian cancer
- breast cancer before the age of 50 on either side of the family (the risk is higher if the relative is your mother or sister)
- relatives with both ovarian and breast cancer
- one or more relatives with two cancers (breast and ovarian, or two types of breast cancer)
- any male relative with breast cancer
- family history of breast or ovarian cancer and Ashkenazi Jewish heritage
- family history of disease associated with hereditary breast cancer, such as Li-Fraunemi or Cowden's syndromes.

The lifetime risk of developing breast cancer among women with altered *BRCA1* or *BRCA2* ranges from 40% to 85%. Mutation in this gene also increases the risk of developing ovarian cancer by 60%. Eastern Europeans with the altered gene have about a 56% increased risk of developing breast cancer.

---

57   G: Syringomyelia

Spinothalamic sensory loss due to compression results in the loss of pain and temperature sensation. However, in dissociated sensory loss the sensation of light touch, which is carried by the posterior column, is intact. There is usually a history of birth trauma, a bony defect, spina bifida, Arnold–Chiari malformation or hydrocephalus associated with this condition.

58 A: Anterior spinal artery thrombosis
A history of valvular heart disease always raises the suspicion of
thromboembolic events. This, together with the presentation of
acute-onset paraplegia, helps you to reach the diagnosis.

59 D: Motor neurone disease
This is a progressive, degenerative condition characterised by
upper and lower motor neurone signs, but no sensory loss. The
three recognised patterns are progressive muscular atrophy,
amyotrophic lateral sclerosis and progressive bulbar palsy.

60 F: Subacute combined degeneration of the cord
The clue lies in the fact that the patient suffers from
malabsorption syndrome. This condition is associated with
pernicious anaemia and poor absorption of vitamin B_{12} from the
gut. The neurological symptoms are of a polyneuropathy,
progressively involving the peripheral nerves and the posterior
and lateral columns of the spinal cord.

61 J: von Recklinghausen's disease
This is also known as 'type 1 neurofibromatosis'. The cutaneous
manifestations are known as *café-au-lait* spots. Associated
abnormalities include phaeochromocytoma, renal artery stenosis,
pulmonary fibrosis, obstructive cardiomyopathy, orbital
haemangioma and fibrous dysplasia of the bone.

---

62 A: Fresh frozen plasma
The best way to achieve warfarin reversal is to give the patient
fresh frozen plasma (and check the INR before any surgical
intervention).

**63 A: A low albumin concentration can indicate cirrhosis or
cancer**
Serum albumin concentrations are indicative of liver synthetic
function, and fall in the presence of chronic liver disease. Low
concentrations are suggestive of underlying cirrhosis or the
development of hepatocellular carcinoma. Cholestasis can be
caused by biliary obstruction (eg gallstones, tumour) or, in the
absence of any physical obstruction, can be associated with drugs

such as erythromycin or chlorpromazine. Cholestasis is typically associated with elevated GGT and ALP levels, whereas hepatocellular injury is characteristically associated with a greater rise in ALT and AST. A number of herbal preparations, including Jamaican bush tea, can cause hepatitis rather than cholestasis. Failure of the prothrombin time to respond to vitamin K indicates impaired liver synthetic function, and is seen in the context of severe hepatocellular impairment, not biliary obstruction.

64   G: Family therapy

Family therapy looks at the interactions within the family and the role that illnesses or particular behaviour plays. In children with behavioural difficulties the problem lies either in the particular condition the child is suffering from or, more commonly, within his/her environment, family or school.

65   I: Psychodynamic psychotherapy

Traditionally, 'I' is the correct answer. However, options C and H are also now accepted by NICE (the National Institute for Clinical Excellence) as first-line therapy (see *NICE guidelines on Eating Disorders*, 2004). Family therapy is recommended for young patients with anorexia nervosa who live with their families.

66   C: Cognitive behaviour therapy

This is one of the most effective psychological interventions, with exposure and response prevention.

67   J: Reality-orientation therapy

'Reality orientation' groups are 'likely to be beneficial', according to available clinical evidence; 'Reminiscent therapy' is also widely practised, although its evidence base for efficacy is 'unknown'. Both therapies are available for elderly people attending day hospitals (see Clinical Evidence, *BMJ*, December 2003).

68   B: Behaviour therapy

This case would involve reinforcing positive behaviour and ignoring unwanted behaviour, as well as modelling, chaining and shaping wanted behaviour.

NB. Analytical psychotherapy, in its classic form, is hardly practised within the NHS. Cognitive behaviour therapy (CBT) and interpersonal therapy (IPT) have the best evidence base for treating depression (see Clinical Evidence, BMJ December 2003).

---

69   **B: It commonly presents with bleeding into muscles and joints**

Haemophilia A is an X-linked recessive condition, characterised by reduced or absent factor VIII activity. Haemophilia B is also an X-linked recessive condition, but is caused by reduced or absent factor IX activity. Because factor IX is more stable than factor VIII, bleeding is generally less severe in those with haemophilia B. Children with haemophilia usually present after the age of 12 months, when they start to walk and suffer more bleeding than would be expected after their inevitable falls. Bleeding is frequently into muscles and joints and leads to crippling arthritis. The PT is normal but the APTT is raised. Bleeding is treated with an intravenous infusion of factor VIII precipitate in people with haemophilia A and of factor IX in those with haemophilia B – recombinant factor concentrates are used because of the risk of viral transmission. Desmopressin infusion is used for minor surgical procedures and dental extraction in people with mild haemophilia because desmopressin stimulates the endogenous release of factor VIII. Haemophilia treatment centres supervise the management of children with bleeding disorders. Families receive support from self-help groups such as The Haemophilia Society.

---

70   **E: SIADH usually occurs due to non-physiological release of ADH from the posterior pituitary or an ectopic source**

SIADH is characterised by hyponatraemia and low serum osmolality, and inappropriately normal-to-high urinary sodium concentrations and osmolarity. It can only be correctly diagnosed in the normovolaemic state and in the absence of diuretic treatment. ADH-secreting tumours are the most common cause of SIADH, but it can also arise as an adverse effect of treatment with opiates, carbamazepine, oxytocin and chlorpropamide. Patients with cardiac failure have increased circulating fluid volumes that arise, in part, through increased ADH secretion. In psychogenic polydipsia, renal function is normal, and ADH concentrations are typically suppressed. Mannitol is an osmotic diuretic, and can be associated with hyponatraemia but SIADH is not a recognised feature. Demeclocycline damages renal ADH effector mechanisms, and can be used as a treatment for SIADH. However, there is a risk of precipitating diabetes insipidus. Addison's disease is associated with mineralocorticoid and glucocorticoid insufficiency.

71 A: Amoebic colitis
The patient has also developed a hepatic abscess, a recognised complication of amoebic colitis. The pus produced has a characteristic anchovy sauce-like appearance.

72 H: Tabes dorsalis
This is a manifestation of tertiary neurosyphilis. This is a complex syndrome in which demyelination of the dorsal roots occur. The features of the syndrome include lightning pains, ataxia, widespread sensory loss and muscular wasting, Charcot's (or neuropathic) joints, Argyll Robertson pupils, ptosis and optic atrophy.

73 C: Mitochondrial myopathy
Most mitochondrial diseases are myopathies and neuropathies and have a maternal pattern of inheritance.

74 D: Myasthenia gravis
This is a disorder of the neuromuscular junction with immune complex-mediated destruction of the acetylcholine receptor. It is associated with other autoimmune conditions, such as thyroid disease, rheumatoid disease, pernicious anaemia and SLE. The proximal limb muscles, muscles of mastication, speech and facial expression are affected initially.

75 A: Dystrophia myotonica
This is inherited as an autosomal dominant condition. Muscle wasting and myotonia are important features of this condition. Frontal balding, atrophy of the testes and the ovary, cardiomyopathy, cataracts, endocrine abnormalities and mental impairment are other features of this disease. Genetic counselling

is vital in such conditions.

76 B: Horner's syndrome

This is due to a lesion of the sympathetic pathway on the same side. In this case it is due to injury to the sympathetic chain during thyroid surgery. It is associated with unilateral pupillary constriction and enophthalmos. There will also be loss of sweating on the same side of the face and the body.

77 B: It is the commonest childhood malignancy

Acute lymphoblastic leukaemia, the most likely diagnosis here, is the commonest childhood malignancy and accounts for 80% of cases of leukaemia in children. The median age of onset is 4years. It has a good prognosis, with an 86% 5-year survival rate. Poor prognostic markers are male gender, black ethnic origin, WCC > 100×10^9/l, age < 1 year or > 10 years, possession of the Philadelphia chromosome, and the persistence of blast cells in the bone marrow at day 28 of treatment. It usually has an insidious onset, with fever, malaise, pallor, infection (sore throat), abnormal bruising, lymphadenopathy and hepatosplenomegaly. Results of blood tests show a low haemoglobin, low platelets, raised/normal/low white cells, and blast cells on the peripheral blood film. A bone marrow examination is essential to confirm the diagnosis. Treatment is with combination chemotherapy.

78 C: In patients with ischaemic heart disease and OSA, nasal CPAP is considered the treatment of choice

Chronic OSA is associated with progressive right heart failure, respiratory acidosis and metabolic alkalosis. Carbonic anhydrase inhibitors, including acetazolamide, can minimise the metabolic consequences associated with sleep apnoea, but are only partially effective and reserved for those with severe metabolic derangement. CPAP is effective in reducing hypercapnia and improving oxygenation, and slows the progression to right heart failure. Weight loss, where appropriate, and intra-oral and intranasal devices are usually sufficient for early management of patients with mild OSA. Uvulopalatopharyngoplasty is effective in a small minority of patients, and is performed only in selected patients with severe OSA.

---

79 G: Phenytoin

80 K: Warfarin

81 A: Alcohol

82 E: Indometacin

83 C: Diethylstilbestrol
Teratogenicity refers to the effects of drugs that can cross the placenta and result in congenital malformations in the fetus. All these answers are self-explanatory; for a more comprehensive list of teratogenic drugs in pregnancy please refer to the *BNF (British National Formulary-Pregnancy Section)*.

---

84 C: Plasma-cell dyscrasia may cause a large volume of protein loss which may not be picked up by dipstick urinalysis
Patients with glomerulonephritis characteristically present with chronic renal impairment, acute nephritis, or nephrotic syndrome, or with asymptomatic proteinuria. There is urinary loss of both albumin and globins, but dipstick urinalysis tests are typically more sensitive to albumin than to other proteins. Dipstick urinalysis can result in false-positive tests due to the normal presence of Tamm–Horsfall glycoprotein. Therefore, a positive test should be confirmed by laboratory urine protein measurement. Normal protein excretion is thought to be up to 100 mg/24 h, including up to 20 mg/l albumin, and dipstick urinalysis tests can normally detect albumin concentrations greater than 150 mg/l. Plasma-cell disorders, including myeloma, are characteristically associated with globulin and Bence Jones protein excretion, and these may not be detected by dipstick analyses.

---

85 C: Fistula-in-ano
Goodsall's rule states that fistulas with external openings posterior to the meridian in the lithotomy position usually curve round to open into the anal canal in the midline posteriorly (following a horseshoe path) and fistulas with anterior external openings open

directly into the anal canal, thus dictating the type of procedure to be performed.

---

86   B: Coarctation of the aorta
In this condition there is localised narrowing of the descending aorta near the ductus arteriosus, usually distal to the left subclavian artery. This results in the formation of collateral vessels which allow the arterial blood to bypass the obstruction to reach the lower part of the body. These collateral vessels become greatly enlarged. As a result, there is enlargement of the left ventricle and heart failure eventually sets in. Associated with Marfan's syndrome, PDA and berry aneurysms.

87   D: Ebstein's anomaly
This is a congenital malposition of the tricuspid valve which may be associated with other cardiac anomalies. The patient may be asymptomatic or symptomatic with cyanosis, triple rhythm, both systolic and diastolic murmurs and heart block.

88   E: Fallot's tetralogy
The two main features of this condition are a large VSD and pulmonary stenosis; over-riding of the aorta and right ventricular hypertrophy are the other features that make up the tetralogy. Progressive cyanosis, initially on exertion and eventually also at rest, is one of the diagnostic signs in this condition.

89   C: Double aortic arch
This congenital anomaly may be asymptomatic in some patients. The symptoms of stridor and dysphagia are secondary to the pressure effects of the aortic arch, which is revealed by the barium swallow.

90   H: Transposition of the great arteries
In this condition the aorta and the pulmonary artery are transpositioned, resulting in the mixing of arterial and venous blood through the fetal channels. Without treatment few babies survive the first year of life.

---

91   A: ASO titre
Rheumatic fever is a systemic illness caused by an abnormal

immune response to group A β-haemolytic *Streptococcus*. It mainly affects children between the ages of 5 and 15 years. There is a latent period of 2–6 weeks following a pharyngeal infection. Diagnosis is made by confirming the presence of two of Jones's major criteria or one major and two minor criteria plus evidence of a preceding streptococcal infection like scarlet fever, and a throat swab growing β-haemolytic *Streptococcus* or a serum ASO titre of > 333 U/l.

Major criteria:
- carditis
- polyarthritis
- erythema marginatum
- subcutaneous nodules
- Sydenham's chorea.

Minor criteria:
- fever
- ESR > 20 mm/h or an elevated C-reactive protein (CRP)
- arthralgia
- prolonged PR interval in the ECG
- previous rheumatic fever or rheumatic heart disease.

---

92   E: There is no increased incidence of viral infections

In health, the spleen removes 'old' platelets from the circulation and protects against infection with capsulated organisms. An early postoperative complication is thrombocythaemia, whereas late complications are due to the increased risks of overwhelming sepsis. Patients should be given pneumococcal vaccine 2 weeks before splenectomy. Asplenic patients should also be considered for vaccination against *Haemophilus influenzae* and meningococci. Routine administration of penicillin is not recommended, but can be considered for selected patients.

---

93   D: DVT

While looking for complications in any postoperative patient, think, 'gastric dilatation on day 3, wound problems on day 5, and PE or DVT on day 10'. When you detect calf tenderness, review the patient carefully as a PE could cost the patient her life.

94   A: Acute tubular necrosis (ATN)

When the patient's BP is stable but their urine output is low, then damage to the kidney has probably already taken place, either pre- or intraoperatively, and measures to prevent further damage need to be put into place.

95 I: Septicaemia

With such a history it most likely that the patient is septic and measures should be put in place to prevent MODS (multiorgan dysfunction syndrome).

96 K: Urinary retention

Retention of urine is a very common presentation after surgery. If the patient appears restless, rule out urinary retention before investigating for other causes, such as pain.

97 A: Acute tubular necrosis (ATN)

Postoperative patients may present with a low urine output, which is usually due to hypovolaemia. The kidneys are the first organs to take the insult, resulting in shutdown, which, with adequate resuscitation, will correct itself. Here, the clue to the development of acute tubular necrosis is the diuresis.

---

98 B: Gum infiltration occurs in the M4 and M5 subtypes

AML is categorised on the basis of the morphological appearance of the bone marrow into seven subsets:

M1 Myeloblastic (no maturation)
M2 Myeloblastic (with maturation)
M3 Promyelocytic
M4 Myelomonocytic
M5 Monoblastic
M6 Erythroblastic
M7 Megakaryoblastic

Gingival hyperplasia due to local infiltration is a characteristic clinical feature of M4 and M5 subtypes. Acute promyelocytic leukaemia (APML, M3) is associated with the risk of DIC. Around 99% of APML patients have a 15:17 chromosomal translocation, which confers a better prognosis after complete remission has been obtained. M6 and M7 subsets predominantly involve red cell and platelet lineages respectively, and are rare.

---

99   D: Tuberculous ulcer

Tuberculous ulcers characteristically have undermined edges.

---

100   D: Pregnant women can safely receive tetanus and diphtheria toxoids

Live attenuated vaccines should generally be avoided in pregnant women, because of risks to the fetus, unless the risks of maternal exposure to infection are sufficiently high to outweigh the potential risks of harm to the fetus. Live attenuated vaccines include measles, rubella and BCG. Inactivated preparations, for example influenza, and detoxified exotoxin vaccines, such as tetanus and diptheria, are comparatively safe.

---

101   E: Anti-Jo-1 antibody

It is important to make the correct diagnosis from the clinical symptoms first, in order to correctly identify the associated autoantibodies. The diagnosis here is dermatomyositis, which is a muscle disorder characterised by necrosis, together with regeneration and inflammation, mainly around the blood vessels. It is characterised by proximal muscle weakness and wasting and the patient typically has difficulty in getting up from a chair. The presence of facial oedema and a purple rash on the face clinches the diagnosis.

102   F: Anti-Ro antibody

The diagnosis here is primary Sjögren's syndrome. The diagnosis is made on the basis of the presence of keratoconjunctivitis sicca (dry eyes) in the absence of rheumatoid arthritis. Dryness of the mouth, skin and vagina may be other associated problems. There are also other systemic associations like arthralgia, Raynaud's phenomenon, other autoimmune disorders, and renal and pulmonary disorders.

103   B: Anticardiolipin antibody

The diagnosis here is antiphospholipid syndrome. Antiphospholipid antibodies affect the platelet membrane and other clotting agents, including protein C, protein S and prothrombin. The main features of this condition are thrombocytopenia, arterial and venous thrombosis, recurrent miscarriages, chorea, migraine, valvular heart disease and atheroma.

104   D: Antihistone antibody   *drug – induced lupus*

The diagnosis here is SLE. The typical photosensitive malar butterfly rash is the clue in this question. The vasculitic lesions are due to Raynaud's disease. Antihistone antibodies are antinuclear antibodies that are present in the majority of patients suffering from this autoimmune vasculitic disorder.

105   G: Anti-Scl-70 antibody

The diagnosis here is systemic sclerosis. There is altered humoral and cell-mediated immunity. Dysphagia is due to oesophageal stricture and there is also associated heartburn, secondary to delayed distal oesophageal peristalsis. The cutaneous manifestations involve skin fibrosis and the tapering of the digits is referred to as 'sclerodactyly'.

106   B: Consider ECT

Transfer to the mother and baby unit is not ideal in this case because of the continuing risk to the baby. Social Services can be informed if there is ongoing concern, even after her admission (eg nobody to look after her and the baby). Remember that electroconvulsive therapy (ECT) provides symptomatic improvement in 80% of depressed patients, compared with around a 66% response to antidepressants. Depressive presentations where ECT is specially indicated include psychomotor retardation and psychotic depression. ECT is also helpful in catatonic schizophrenia, and can be beneficial in mania and resistant schizophrenia (but is rarely used here). However, improvements are not sustained after ECT discontinuation. Treatment usually comprises 6–12 sessions, and patients are reviewed regularly. Patient consent should ideally be obtained by the consultant (RMO, responsible medical officer) and before every session. However, ECT can be given without consent providing there are two medical recommendations. Mortality is comparable to that for minor operative procedures. The main side-effects of ECT include headache and brief confusion on recovery. A longer term, retrograde memory loss sometimes occurs and adds to the controversy regarding ECT; a poor response to ECT is also associated with memory difficulties. It can be delivered either unilaterally (less efficacious and better tolerated) to the non-dominant side (mostly the right) or bilaterally.

107 C: Toxic shock syndrome

Toxic shock syndrome usually occurs in the setting of staphylococcal infection of skin or soft tissues, and is mediated by the endotoxin TSS-1. Characteristic clinical features also include hypotension, shock and very high body temperatures (> 39.5°C). Treatment is predominantly with supportive care to ensure adequate circulating volume, administration of pressor agents to maintain systemic blood pressure, and antibiotic treatment.

108 A: DiGeorge syndrome

This syndrome is caused by deletion of chromosome 22. The clinical features are developmental delay, a short philtrum, a thin upper lip and prominent ears. Other features are hypocalcaemia and T-cell deficiency. Congenital heart defects common in this condition are interrupted aortic arch and VSD.

109 I: Prader–Willi syndrome

This syndrome is caused by a deletion of chromosome 15. The clinical features are hypotonia, obesity, hypogonadism and developmental delay. Affected children have a thin upper lip, a narrow face, almond-shaped eyes and down-turned lips.

110 D: Fragile X syndrome

Fragile X syndrome is inherited as an X-linked recessive disorder. Clinical features are moderate learning difficulties, macrocephaly, macro-orchidism, and characteristic facies – a long face, large everted ears, a prominent mandible and a large forehead.

111 E: Klinefelter's syndrome

This syndrome has a 47,XXY genotype. The clinical features are hypogonadism, infertility, tall stature and gynaecomastia. Intelligence is usually normal but affected individuals may have educational and psychological problems.

112 H: Pierre Robin syndrome

Inheritance pattern: most are sporadic; some may be due to Stickler's syndrome, which has autosomal dominant inheritance. The clinical features are micrognathia, glossoptosis, cleft palate and feeding difficulties.

NB. Use any standard book to read about all the genetic disorders described in the answers above, and others, as questions commonly come up in the exams.

---

113 B: Intravenous β-blockers are the agents of choice

Aortic dissection involves shearing of the medial and intimal vascular layers, and is more prevalent among patients with long-standing hypertension and those with pre-existing atherosclerotic vascular disease. Complications of thoracic aortic dissection include aortic valve incompetence, coronary and subclavian arterial occlusion, acute cardiac failure, and leakage causing haemopericardium and haemothorax. Blood pressure should be adequately controlled as soon as possible so as to reduce extension of the dissection, and β-blockers are regarded as the treatment of choice. Venodilators, and direct arterial vasodilators such as diazoxide, are more difficult to titrate to blood pressure response, and are associated with an increased risk of hypotension. Emergency surgery is required for many aortic dissections, and the 10-year survival rate varies from 20% to 60%.

---

114 E: Ramstedt's operation

Ramstedt's operation is a pyloromyotomy.

---

115 C: Glucose tolerance test

Once again, it is important to make the correct diagnosis from the clinical symptoms described, in order to choose the most suitable investigation. The diagnosis here is acromegaly, secondary to excess growth hormone secretion from a pituitary tumour. The symptoms described are diagnostic. Acromegalic patients show a diabetic glucose tolerance test.

116   K: Short Synacthen® test
The diagnosis here is Addison's disease. Tuberculosis is the second commonest cause of destruction of the adrenal cortex after autoimmune disorders. The classic symptoms of postural hypotension and oral pigmentation help to clinch the diagnosis.

117   B: Dexamethasone suppression test
Here the diagnosis is Cushing's syndrome. Patients with Cushing's syndrome fail to suppress plasma or urinary cortisol.

118   D: High/normal urine osmolality with low serum osmolality
The diagnosis here is SIADH (syndrome of inappropriate ADH secretion) and this is secondary to increased ectopic production seen in lung cancer (commonly small cell carcinoma of the lung). The symptoms are usually vague, with confusion, fits, irritability and coma. The symptoms are due to excessive water retention and continued sodium excretion, which result in dilutional hyponatraemia.

119   H: Increased serum 17-Hydroxyprogesterone
Here the diagnosis is congenital adrenal hyperplasia (CAH). This is an autosomal recessive condition caused by the deficiency of an enzyme in the cortisol synthesis pathway, most commonly a deficiency of 21-hydroxylase. Due to the decreased cortisol synthesis, there is an increase in ACTH secretion, which in turn leads to diversion of steroid precursors to produce more androgens. Short stature and hirsutism before the menarche are diagnostic features.

---

120   D: Mefenamic acid and tranexamic acid
This is the first line of management for primary menorrhagia. Although the cause for the menorrhagia needs to be investigated, this is the recommended treatment in the first

instance. The dosage is tranexamic acid 1 g tid/qds and
mefenamic acid 500 mg tid, during the periods.

---

121   A: Flow volume loop

In extrathoracic airway obstruction, there is often limitation of
the inspiratory flow rate and, to a lesser extent, the expiratory
flow rate. The flow curves are flattened compared with normal,
and overall vital capacity is reduced. Spirometry will typically be
reduced, but this is a very non-specific test, and will not assist
diagnosis. Slow vital capacity measurement can be used to give a
more accurate measure of vital capacity than forced measures in
patients with severe chronic obstructive pulmonary disease.
Transfer factor is largely a measure of gas exchange at alveolar
level, and will normally be preserved. Mouth pressure
measurements have no diagnostic role.

---

122   E: Rapidly proliferative glomerulonephritis (RPGN)

RPGN, also known as 'crescentic glomerulonephritis', based on
its microscopic morphology, is associated with rapid decline in
renal function and the need for renal replacement therapy. It
occurs in immune-complex nephritis, and is seen in patients
with polyarteritis nodosa, Wegener's granulomatosis and
Goodpasture's syndrome. The pattern of crescentic glomerular
involvement in the context of sinusitis and diffuse pulmonary
infiltrates is strongly suggestive of Wegener's granulomatosis,
and the diagnosis can be confirmed by a positive c-ANCA
immunofluorescence test.

---

123   C: Agoraphobia

Agoraphobia is a condition characterised by anxiety and
avoidance of crowds, public places, and travelling away from
home or alone.

124   J: Post-traumatic stress disorder

Post-traumatic stress disorder arises following exposure to a
threatening situation, which is then followed by 'reliving'
symptoms (flashbacks and nightmares), hypervigilance,
insomnia, emotional numbing and avoidance.

125   E: Generalised anxiety state
Generalised anxiety disorder is characterised by generalised,
free-floating and persistent anxiety.

126   A: Abnormal bereavement reaction
An abnormal bereavement reaction is associated with a chronic
course (6months), and it may or may not be associated
with depression. Often, there are suicidal thoughts,
pseudohallucinations, mummification of articles of the dead and
avoidance of reminders of death. The risk of abnormal grief
increases if there was a dependent or ambivalent relationship, or
when normal emotional expression of grief is not possible.
'Guided mourning' with a counsellor or psychotherapist is often
thought to be helpful. It is included under 'Adjustment disorder'
in ICD-10.

127   H: Obsessive-compulsive disorder
Obsessions are recurrent, unpleasant thoughts, which are
unsuccessfully resisted. The person experiencing them
appreciates, to some extent, that they are unusual and that they
are their own thoughts. Compulsions are ritualistic behaviours
or thoughts that often accompany obsessions.

---

128   D: Midline
A midline incision is performed to gain access to the
retroperitoneal structures and the organs are retracted with the
help of retractors to expose the lymph nodes for dissection.

---

129   E: Constrictive pericarditis
The *y* wave in the JVP is due to the opening of the tricuspid
valve at the end of ventricular systole. However, in constrictive
pericarditis the stiff ventricular walls cannot be easily distended,
causing a rise in the venous pressure after the initial fall. This
rapid fall and then rise of the JVP is known as 'Friedreich's sign'.
This is also seen in tricuspid regurgitation.

130   A: Budd–Chiari syndrome
This is a veno-occlusive condition seen in hypercoagulable states
causing occlusion of the hepatic vein and hence obstructing the
venous return. Other causes include abdominal tumours, the

contraceptive pill, hepatic cell carcinoma, and radiotherapy or trauma to the liver.

131   G: Meigs' syndrome
This condition is associated with a benign ovarian fibroma or a thecoma. Ascites and pleural effusion are two of its features.

132   C: Chylous ascites
This is due to obstruction of the main lymphatic duct by malignant cells. The increased triglyceride is due to the presence of chylomicrons.

133   I: Tuberculous peritonitis
This is one of the commonest opportunistic infections among HIV-positive patients.

---

134   B: Cervical incompetence
The most common cause for recurrent painless fetal loss in the second trimester is cervical incompetence. The other options explain recurrent early fetal loss in the first trimester. The diagnosis is usually made by a finding of cervical funnelling on the transvaginal scan. The treatment is preventive – a cervical suture is put in at 14–16 weeks of pregnancy. This is usually removed between 36 weeks and 37 weeks of pregnancy, before the onset of labour.

---

135   C: HbsAg-negative, anti-HBs-positive, anti-HBc-negative, anti-Hbe-negative
HBsAg (surface antigen) is sought as initial confirmation of acute hepatitis B infection; in certain cases, it can be cleared rapidly, and IgM anti-HBc antibodies (anti-core antigen antibodies) are a helpful confirmatory test. Hepatitis B viral DNA is a highly sensitive test of viral replication, and determined by PCR techniques. Anti-HBs (anti-surface antigen antibodies) are a useful indicator of immunity due to prior infection (anti-Hbe-positive) or vaccination (anti-Hbe-negative), and can take several months to develop full immunity. Titres of anti-HBs are used to determine the adequacy of immunity and the need for further vaccination boosters.

---

136 D: Gout
   Gout can occur even with a normal uric acid level.

137 I: Rheumatoid arthritis
   Remember the sites of involvement – the proximal
   interphalangeal and metacarpophalangeal joints of the hands,
   the wrists, elbows, shoulders, cervical spine, knees, ankles and
   the small joints of the feet.

138 K: Tennis elbow
   Remember: the 't' in 'lateral' stands for 'tennis'.

139 H: Psoriatic arthritis
   The involvement of distal joints associated with red scaly
   patches of skin is an indication of psoriatic arthropathy.

140 F: Osteoarthritis
   Elderly patients with walking difficulties are usually suffering
   from osteoarthritis.

---

141 D: The seizure frequency would be most likely to increase
   during pregnancy
   Assuming that the mother continues to receive the usual
   phenytoin dose during pregnancy, seizure frequency would be
   expected to remain the same. Changes in extracellular fluid
   volume and albumin concentrations mean that the circulating
   phenytoin concentrations would be expected to fall slightly; the
   proportion of free unbound drug would increase, however, so
   that overall free drug concentrations remain the same or
   increase slightly. Although there is a recognised risk of fetal
   abnormalities due to anti-epileptic treatment, this risk is
   outweighed by the benefits, to both mother and fetus, of
   remaining seizure-free on treatment.

---

142 B: Serum calcium
   The serum calcium should be measured to check for
   hypocalcaemia as the parathyroid gland may be removed
   inadvertently during this procedure.

---

143   **C: Neuropathic joint disease**
Neuropathic joint disease can, as in this scenario, be very destructive and reach an advanced stage before coming to medical attention. The basis for the condition is loss of pressure and pain sensation at the involved site. Crepitus is a characteristic sign of erosive and destructive local bony changes at the joint margins.

144   **A: Chromium deficiency**
Chromium deficiency results in glucose intolerance.

145   **I: Selenium deficiency**
This results in Keshan disease, which is encountered in parts of China. This trace element is a vital component of the glutathione peroxidase enzyme, which plays an important role in the body defence mechanism protecting cells against lipid peroxidation. Its actions are synergistic with those of vitamin E. It is also thought to be important for maintaining sperm mitochondria.

146   **J: Zinc deficiency**
Zinc is important for the actions of DNA and RNA polymerase. It acts as an antiviral, antifungal and antibacterial agent. It is also important for the actions of a host of hormones, including thyroid hormones, glucagon, insulin, growth hormone and the sex hormones. It also helps in brain development, especially of the hippocampal region.

147   **G: Molybdenum deficiency**
Molybdenum is important for the action of xanthine oxidase, which helps in the degradation of purines and the production of uric acid. Its deficiency therefore causes hypouricaemia.

148   **E: Iodine deficiency**
The geographical origin of the patient is an important clue to the answer. People in hilly areas have an endemic deficiency of iodine in their diet. They may be asymptomatic or symptomatic, depending on the severity of the deficiency.

149   D: Regular slit-lamp examination should be performed

JCA occurs in three characteristic patterns: Still's disease, juvenile rheumatoid arthritis and juvenile ankylosing spondylitis. Still's disease is the most common of these, and rheumatoid factor is usually negative. It can manifest with systemic features (typically in children under 5 years old), such as fever, lymphadenopathy and rash, and arthritis might be a minor feature of the condition. An oligoarticular form of Still's disease typically affects up to four large joints in children aged 10–15 years, and is frequently associated with iritis. The risk of iritis is greatest in those with raised antinuclear antibody titres, and regular slit-lamp examination is required to detect this potential complication, which can result in blindness. A polyarticular form of Still's disease can occur, and is symmetrical, though involvement of the small joints is less common than in rheumatoid arthritis.

150   E: Young maternal age

Sudden infant death syndrome (SIDS) is the sudden death of a baby where no cause can be found after full investigation and autopsy. Established risk factors are:

- prone sleeping position
- parental smoking
- male infant
- previous SIDS in the family
- winter
- overheating
- young maternal age
- poverty, low socioeconomic class
- preceding respiratory infection
- high parity.

151   J: Organophosphates

The clue lies in the reference to the SLUD response, an acronym that stands for salivation, lacrimation, urination and diarrhoea. Organophosphate insecticides inactivate cholinesterase. Other signs to look for are constricted pupils, muscle fasciculations, coma and respiratory failure.

152 G: Lithium
The ECG changes are due to electrolyte imbalance, such as
hypokalaemia. Lithium overdose can occur accidentally in
people who are on antipsychotics, in whom the additional use of
diuretics causes impaired lithium elimination by the kidney.
Treatment includes increased hydration and, in severe cases,
peritoneal dialysis or haemodialysis may be necessary.

153 A: Arsenic
The fact that this person is in the spraying industry gives a clue
regarding the source of poisoning. The typical pigmentation of
the skin is referred to as the 'raindrop' sign.

154 H: Mercury
This is also a heavy metal like arsenic. The tremors seen in
mercury poisoning are referred to as the 'hatters shakes'.
Treatment involves the administration of dimercaprol or
penicillamine.

155 F: Lead
This is a notifiable occupational disease in this country.
Basophilic stippling is seen in the peripheral blood film in these
patients. Peripheral nerve lesions include foot drop and wrist
drop. Treatment includes administration of calcium EDTA,
D-penicillamine or dimercaprol.

---

156 D: Leave alone
A foreign body that has passed into the stomach should come
out with the faeces – it is expected that if something has passed
through the oesophagus, then it should be able to pass though
the rest of the bowel unless it is spiky (eg an open safety pin).
The parents should be reassured and asked to monitor the
child's faeces to check that it has been passed.

**157 B: Colchicine gives effective pain relief but is frequently
associated with profuse diarrhoea**
Acute gout becomes more likely with advancing age, and is due
to inflammation at the site of preformed urate crystals within
large and medium-sized joints. It is significantly more common

in patients receiving thiazide diuretics and thromboprophylactic doses of aspirin. A sudden increase or decrease in serum urate concentrations can provoke acute gout, and allopurinol treatment is usually reserved until the acute episode has resolved. Colchicine gives effective analgesia and has anti-inflammatory effects, but dose escalation is often limited by gastrointestinal symptoms. Serum urate concentrations are only poorly associated with the risks of acute gout, and do not confirm or refute the diagnosis. Acute gout is more likely in patients with active psoriasis due to increased cell turnover and purine metabolism.

---

158   C: Orchidopexy reduces chances of later malignancy

At birth, 5% of full-term male infants have an undescended testis; the incidence is higher in preterm infants. The testicles continue to descend, and by 3months 1.5% of boys will have an undescended testis, with little change thereafter. Surgical placement of the undescended testis into the scrotum (orchidopexy) is performed during the second year of life to optimise the child's reproductive potential. Fertility after orchidopexy for a unilaterally undescended testis is close to normal, but bilateral undescended testes leads to sterility. Undescended testicles have a histological abnormality and are at an increased risk of malignancy, but there is evidence showing that early orchidopexy reduces this risk. Treatment with intranasal gonadotrophin-releasing hormone has been unreliable.

---

159   C: Detrusor overactivity (DO)

Detrusor overactivity was previously also known as 'detrusor instability'. The symptoms described here are typically seen in women with an overactive bladder, which results in urge incontinence. The diagnosis is clinched by performing urodynamic studies. It is caused by the bladder contracting spontaneously, with or without provocation. Overexcitability of the detrusor muscle and reduced motor innervation of the bladder wall are two of the factors that have been said to be responsible. Treatment involves taking anticholinergic drugs and training in bladder drill.

160   B: Cystocele

Although you may think that option D (genuine stress incontinence) is the right answer to this question, the clinical findings described in the second half of the question rule out that possibility. Approximately 50% of patients with stress incontinence also have a cystocele. Childbirth with damage to the pelvic floor due to long labour, large babies and instrumental deliveries are some of the aetiological factors. Mild symptoms can be treated with pelvic floor exercises while moderate to severe cystocele is managed either with surgery in the younger patient or with a pessary in elderly patients who are not suitable for surgery.

161   K: Vesico-vaginal fistula

The history of having had an instrumental delivery 3 weeks before is the clue in this question. This is an important medicolegal issue and needs to be managed appropriately. Once the diagnosis is confirmed, the patient needs to be seen by the consultant who she was booked under for antenatal care. It is important to involve the most senior clinician right at the onset in order to address the potentially complicated medicolegal issues. The patient needs to be properly debriefed about her intrapartum management and advised of the long-term implications. The patient should then be referred to a urogynaecologist who specialises in the management of such problems.

162   E: Interstitial cystitis

This is also known as 'non-bacterial cystitis'. This could be due to a leak in the bladder wall, causing urine to leak in and cause pancystitis. The symptoms are usually increased frequency, depending on toilet availability, nocturia, and a feeling of incomplete emptying. The patient is generally very miserable and anxious and has constant or recurrent symptoms. Cystoscopy and bladder wall biopsy may be helpful in diagnosis. The treatment is mainly supportive, with measures such as teaching bladder drill, prolonged antibiotic prophylaxis, small doses of steroids and the raising of urinary pH with potassium citrate.

163 F: Procidentia

This is once again a typical presentation in the elderly. When the whole uterus with the cervix lies outside the vagina it is called 'procidentia'. It is also associated with decubitus ulcers (dependent ulcers) and the vaginal mucosa becomes dry and keratinised, causing bleeding and irritation. The ulcers may get infected and present with foul-smelling discharge. Treatment in the elderly is by reducing the procidentia and packing the vagina with roller gauze soaked in antiseptic cream till the ulcers heal. If infection is present you can also prescribe systemic antibiotics. Long-term treatment in those who are not fit for surgery is with a pessary. A shelf pessary is ideal in those with a large procidentia. These patients may also need long-term catheterisation to prevent retention of urine due to the mechanical obstruction caused by the prolapsed uterus.

164 B: Aspirin

With the exception of paracetamol, all of these drugs are highly protein-bound, and are excreted in breast milk in comparatively small quantities. Aspirin, even in small quantities, can have significant anti-platelet effects in the newborn because the immature platelets are more sensitive to the effects of cyclo-oxygenase inhibition. Furthermore, aspirin increases the risk of Reye's syndrome in all children, potentially up to the age of 16 years. This is an idiosyncratic reaction that is not dependent on the dose or duration of aspirin exposure. Paracetamol taken in therapeutic doses is excreted in small amounts in breast milk, and would not be expected to have any adverse consequences in the newborn.

165 D: 85% of expected weight for age and height

This criterion is agreed upon in both the ICD-10 and the DSM-4. Alternatively, body mass index (BMI) can be assessed, (weight in kg per height in metres squared, kg/m^2). A BMI of less than 17.5 is an alternative indication for the diagnosis, along with a fear of weight gain, body image distortion and an active pursuit of weight loss. Apart from dieting, recognised weight loss techniques include over-exercising and the misuse of laxatives, purgatives, diuretics and appetite suppressants.

166   B: Co-codamol

Reduced conscious level, shallow respirations and cardiovascular instability could all be accounted for by an overdose of amitriptyline (a tricyclic antidepressant), diazepam or the codeine component of co-codamol. Pinpoint pupils strongly suggests opiate effects, whereas tricyclic antidepressants typically cause mydriasis, and benzodiazepines have little effect on pupil size. Ecstasy would be more likely to cause agitation, restlessness, and dilated pupils, rather than reduced conscious level. Ibuprofen is unlikely to alter conscious level in the absence of severe intoxication, and does not cause miosis. Treatment of this woman should involve administration of naloxone, ventilatory support (if required), and consideration of paracetamol concentration at 4 hours post-ingestion.

---

167   A: Left frontal cortex

The theory of cerebral dominance is important to analyse this situation. Almost all right-handed individuals have language function in the left hemisphere and so a cerebral event in this hemisphere will result in dysphasia, agraphia and acquired dyslexia.

168   B: Left parietal region

A lesion in this region results in constructional apraxia, right-left disorientation, homonymous field defects, and failure to recognise the surroundings.

169   F: Right temporal region

These features are associated with lesions in this area of the brain.

170   G: Occipital region

Visuospatial defects and disturbance in visual recognition are classic signs associated with occipital lesions.

171   C: Left temporoparietal region

This is also known as 'Wernicke's aphasia'.

---

172   A: Basal cell carcinoma
Basal cell carcinomas are seen in the cheek area above the line joining the angle of the mouth and the tragus.

---

173   A: Base of skull fracture
The signs of a basal skull fracture are 'racoon' eyes, the battle sign (bruising over the mastoid process), rhinorrhoea, otorrhoea and haemotympanum.

174   D: Extradural haemorrhage
A lucid interval is suggestive of an extradural haemorrhage.

175   J: Subdural haemorrhage
Falls in elderly people tend to result in subdural haemorrhages.

176   B: Concussion
This is a mild presentation of head injury and no further management is required.

177   E: Intracerebral haemorrhage
This is a severe presentation of head injury. Such patients need immediate resuscitation and the involvement of a neurosurgeon.

---

178   A: DC cardioversion
In the setting of ventricular tachycardia with haemodynamic compromise, or ventricular fibrillation, immediate DC cardioversion is the key priority. Thereafter, cardiopulmonary resuscitation should be commenced, and intravenous access established for administration of adrenaline (epinephrine). Amiodarone should be considered in certain situations, and might make DC cardioversion attempts more successful. Adenosine is appropriate only for diagnosis or termination of SVT. Beta-blocker treatment would be detrimental in the above scenario because it would compromise blood pressure further, and antagonise the effects of adrenaline.

---

179   C: Ovarian thecoma
The clue to the correct answer lies in the phrase 'sudden onset of hirsutism'. This usually implies a sudden massive increase in

testosterone levels due to a testosterone-secreting tumour that may arise either from the adrenals or from the ovary. The testosterone levels are usually up to three times the normal limit in PCOS. The fact that the U&Es are normal, together with the symptoms of sudden baldness and secondary amenorrhoea point more towards an ovarian cause than to the adrenals.

180   C: Familial Mediterranean fever
This is a condition of unknown aetiology, classically seen among Jews and Arabs. Recurrent attacks may be prevented by the use of colchicine.

181   D: Kawasaki disease
Infection is the underlying cause for this condition. There is associated vasculitis that can affect the coronary arteries, resulting in acquired heart disease in children. Plasma exchange and administration of gammaglobulin are the main modalities of treatment.

182   H: Q fever
This is caused by *Coxiella burnetii*, a rickettsial organism. Sheep, cattle and other farm animals are the primary reservoir of this organism. Ticks are the intermediate hosts. Humans usually become infected after inhalation of aerosols or when they come in direct contact with infected animal products. The infection usually resolves by itself but administration of doxycycline usually reduces the duration of the fever. Tetracycline, rifampicin, co-trimoxazole and linomycin are some of the other antibiotics used.

183   G: Polyarteritis nodosa
This is a vasculitic disorder causing aneurysms in medium-sized arteries. Diagnosis is usually made on renal or mesenteric vessel angiography.

184   B: EBV infection
This is also called 'glandular fever' or 'infectious mononucleosis'. The heterophil antibody test, also known as the

'Paul-Bunnell test', is positive. Treatment is usually supportive and, rarely, steroids are used in extreme cases.

---

185   A: 1% burn

According to the 'rule of nine', any burn involving the palm is considered to be a 1% burn.

---

186   B: Intravenous 1.26% sodium bicarbonate at 250 ml/h

The clinical scenario suggests a possible stroke, on the basis of the left hemiparesis. The investigations indicate renal impairment, and the bruising suggests that the raised CK can be accounted for by skeletal rather than cardiac muscle damage. In this situation, aspirin and streptokinase are unlikely to offer any immediate benefit and could even be hazardous. The high serum urate concentration is consistent with rhabdomyolysis. In this scenario, a secure airway should be maintained and ventilatory support given if needed. The patient should be given intravenous fluids for rehydration, with careful monitoring of central venous pressure and urine output. Dialysis might be required if conservative measures alone are inadequate. Urinary alkalinisation appears to reduce renal injury in the setting of rhabdomyolysis, and saline might be preferred to dextrose as a crystalloid for rehydration.

---

187   F: Sickle cell disease (HbS)

The homozygous state (SS) results from inheritance of two β-globin genes in which there is a single amino acid substitution (glutamine for valine) on codon6 of the β chain. Commonly seen in people of African, Mediterranean or Middle-Eastern origin, this does not lead to a clinical problem in itself. When these haemoglobin molecules are exposed to the deoxgenated state, however, they become rigid and the red cells assume a sickle shape. These sickled red cells have a shortened lifespan and become trapped in the microcirculation, resulting in thrombosis and ischaemia. Low oxygen, dehydration and cold all lead to sickling. Clinical manifestations include: moderate anaemia (6–8 g/dl) with jaundice from haemolysis; hand-foot syndrome in late infancy, in which there is swelling and pain in the fingers and toes due to vaso-occlusion; autosplenectomy due to splenic infarction; increased risk of sepsis; and priapism. Other features are short stature, delayed puberty, cardiac enlargement and renal dysfunction resulting from chronic anaemia, gallstones due to excess bilirubin excretion, and leg ulcers. Management includes hydration, oxygenation and warmth during acute crises, and analgesia for pain relief. Blood transfusion may be required during aplastic sequestration or haemolytic crisis.

188   G: Thalassaemia

This is caused by a deficiency in the production of the β chains of haemoglobin. Gamma chain synthesis continues beyond infancy, leading to an increase in HbF, and increased β-chain production, which leads to an increase in the amount of HbA$_2$. Commonly seen in people from the Mediterranean and Middle East. Clinical features include: pallor, jaundice, maxillary overgrowth, frontal bossing of the skull and splenomegaly. Patients require multiple blood transfusions. The aim of treatment is to maintain the haemoglobin concentration above 10 g/dl to reduce growth retardation. Repeated transfusion leads to iron overload and subsequent tissue damage. Chelating agents are used to increase iron excretion. Bone marrow transplant is curative but is limited to children who have an HLA-matched, compatible sibling donor.

189   B: G6PD deficiency

This is the most common enzyme deficiency, and transmission is X-linked recessive. It is common in Mediterranean, Middle Eastern, Oriental and Afro-Carribean populations. G6PD is a rate-limiting enzyme in the hexose monophosphate shunt which maintains glutathione in a reduced state, and prevents oxidative damage of red cells. G6PD deficiency leads to oxidant-induced haemolysis. The condition is characterised by episodes of haemolysis rather than a chronic haemolytic state. Clinical features include: neonatal jaundice (onset within the first 3 days of life), episodes of drug- or infection-induced jaundice, and favism (in which the ingestion of broad beans causes haemolysis). Haemolysis presents with fever, malaise, passage of dark urine (as it contains haemoglobin and urobilinogen) and a rapid fall in haemoglobin. Drugs which cause haemolysis include ciprofloxacin, primaquine, nalidixic acid, nitrofurantoin, co-trimoxazole and dapsone. Parents should be provided with a list of drugs to avoid and the symptoms should be explained to them (pallor, jaundice and dark urine). Blood transfusion may be needed in acute haemolysis.

190   D: Iron deficiency anaemia

Iron deficiency in infants is commonly due to poor dietary intake. In infants it is commonly due to lack of breast-feeding, delayed introduction of solids and early introduction of pasteurised milk. Young children have a much higher iron requirement than adults. A 1-year-old infant requires 8 mg of iron a day. The clinical features are pallor, tiredness and pica (eating of non-food material such as chalk or gravel). It is associated with behavioural and intellectual deficiency. Diagnosis is by blood count, which shows a low haemoglobin, and blood film which shows a microcytic hypochromic anaemia. Children often have low iron stores and develop anaemia later on. In suspected deficiency, the ferritin level should be checked. Management involves dietary advice and supplementation of iron. Children should be investigated to rule out other causes for iron deficiency, such as a haemolytic disorder, coeliac disease or Crohn's disease.

---

191   E: N-acetylcysteine infusion should be commenced and LFTs checked at 24 hours

After acute paracetamol ingestion, serum concentrations reach peak levels at 1–3 hours, then fall rapidly, and may be undetectable beyond 18–24 hours. With staggered overdoses and late presentation after overdose, blood levels are a less reliable indicator of the need for N-acetylcysteine treatment. Ingestion of more than 150 mg/kg over 24 hours, as in this scenario, can be associated with hepatocellular damage, and N-acetylcysteine should be commenced. Deranged baseline LFTs indicate patients at higher risk of liver impairment. Even if LFTs and the prothrombin time are normal at presentation, N-acetylcysteine administration should be continued, and blood tests rechecked 24 hours later (around 48 hours post-ingestion) to exclude significant liver damage.

---

192   C: Gender identity disorder

This presentation is typical of gender identity disorder of childhood. If the difficulty is pervasive it may present as transsexualism, but in many cases it does resolve. Transvestism, on the other hand, is merely cross-dressing. Fetishism is associated with the obtaining of sexual arousal from an inanimate object.

---

193   G: Perindopril

This is an ACE inhibitor which, by lowering systemic vascular resistance, reducing venous pressure and reducing the circulating levels of catecholamines, effectively improves myocardial performance. Although these drugs act on the ACE (and therefore on the renin-angiotensin mechanism), they can act even when plasma renin activity is normal.

194   B: Atenolol

This reduces early mortality in the acute phase and has a protective effect when used in the convalescent period.

195   I: Sodium nitroprusside

This is a vasodilating agent which is very useful for achieving controlled hypotension during anaesthesia.

196   F: Moxonidine

This is a centrally acting antihypertensive drug used in treating mild to moderate essential hypertension.

197   E: Losartan

This is a specific angiotensin II-receptor antagonist, which has properties similar to ACE inhibitors. However, unlike ACE inhibitors, it does not prevent the degradation of kinins and hence does not cause the persistent dry cough that is associated with ACE inhibitors.

---

198 **D: Day 21 progesterone level**

This is the easiest test to use to check her ovulatory status. If day 21 progesterone results are more than 30 nmol/l in two cycles, then the patient is ovulating.

---

199 **A: Bumetanide**

Diuretic treatment has more profound haemodynamic effects in elderly than young patients, due to diminished compensatory mechanisms of fluid homeostasis. Other drugs that require particular caution in elderly patients are those cleared by renal elimination, due to impaired renal blood flow, including digoxin and metformin. ACE inhibitors and NSAIDs are more likely to be nephrotoxic in elderly patients, due to diminished renal blood flow, and more likely to precipitate renal impairment. Sedative drugs are likely to have greater effects in elderly patients because of higher CNS concentrations attained in the presence of a less effective blood-brain barrier mechanism.

---

200 **A: ASA 1**

'ASA 1' means that the patient is normal and fit and 'ASA 5' would mean that the patient is moribund and not fit for surgery.

Index

The EMQs and SBAs are indexed separately, by question number. The key is as follows:
M – Medicine; S – Surgery; OG – Obstetrics & Gynaecology; PA – Paediatrics; PS – Psychiatry; PR – Practice Paper.

Extended matching question index

Single best answer index